A Life of Healing

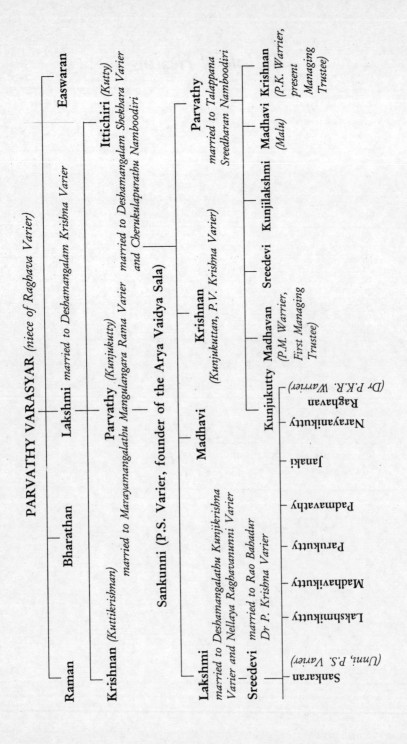

PARVATHY VARASYAR (niece of Raghava Varier)

Raman **Bharathan** **Lakshmi** *married to Deshamangalam Krishna Varier* **Easwaran**

Krishnan *(Kuttikrishnan)*

Parvathy *(Kunjukutty)*
married to Marayamangalathu Mangulangara Rama Varier

Ittichiri *(Kutty)*
married to Deshamangalam Shekhara Varier and Cherukulapurathu Namboodiri

Sankunni (P.S. Varier, founder of the Arya Vaidya Sala)

Lakshmi
married to Deshamangalathu Kunjikrishna Varier and Nellaya Raghavanunni Varier

Madhavi

Krishnan
(Kunjukuttan, P.V. Krishna Varier)

Parvathy
married to Talappana Sreedharan Namboodiri

Sreedevi *married to Rao Bahadur Dr P. Krishna Varier*

Sankaran
(Unni, P.S. Varier) | **Lakshmikutty** | **Madhavikutty** | **Parukutty** | **Padmavathy** | **Janaki** | **Narayanikutty** | **Raghavan**
(Dr P.K.R. Warier)

Kunjukutty **Madhavan**
(P.M. Warier, First Managing Trustee)

Sreedevi **Kunjilakshmi** **Madhavi** **Krishnan**
(P.K. Warier, present Managing Trustee)
(Malu)

A LIFE OF HEALING

A Biography of
Vaidyaratnam P.S. Varier

Gita Krishnankutty

VIKING

VIKING
Penguin Books India (P) Ltd., 11 Community Centre, Panchsheel Park, New Delhi 110 017, India
Penguin Books Ltd., 80 Strand, London WC2R 0RL, UK
Penguin Putnam Inc., 375 Hudson Street, New York, NY 10014, USA
Penguin Books Australia Ltd., Ringwood, Victoria, Australia
Penguin Books Canada Ltd., 10 Alcorn Avenue, Suite 300, Toronto, Ontario, M4V 3B2, Canada
Penguin Books (NZ) Ltd., Cnr Rosedale and Airborne Roads, Albany, Auckland, New Zealand

First published in Viking by Penguin Books India 2001

Copyright © Vaidyaratnam P.S. Varier's Arya Vaidya Sala, Kottakkal 2001

10 9 8 7 6 5 4 3 2 1

Typeset in Garamond by SÜRYA, New Delhi
Printed at Chaman Offset Printers, New Delhi

Contents

Acknowledgements

I would like to express my gratitude to all the people at the Arya Vaidya Sala, Kottakkal, who generously gave me so much of their time and extended valuable help to me in preparing this book.

Foreword

Ayurveda has won universal recognition. Its holistic approach and healing effects have been widely acclaimed. But this was not the case a century ago when Vaidyaratnam P.S. Varier founded the Arya Vaidya Sala in 1902. The age-old tradition of indigenous medicine was under severe attack from several quarters. The colonial masters, in their eagerness to assert the superiority of western science, condemned native values and did all they could to delegitimize the authenticity of Indian systems of medicines. The system had internal weaknesses too: stagnant knowledge, ignorant practitioners and non-availability of quality medicines. Thus the Ayurvedic system of treatment was on the verge of extinction at the beginning of the last century.

What P.S. Varier did to retrieve the lost glory to Ayurveda is part of history now. He organized his fellow-physicians, instilled confidence in them and led them to a 'creative introspection' based on their own experience. Himself a 'critical insider', he could, with their help, rejuvenate the system by integrating it with western epistemology. He introduced systematic study of Ayurveda by his pioneering institutional efforts, disseminated the ancient wisdom through scientific publications and ensured the quality of medicines by adopting modern techniques of manufacturing. His activities were not confined to the medical field. As a good physician, scholar, poet, dramatist, musician, entrepreneur and philanthropist, his efforts embraced the entire realm of our cultural life. P.S. Varier was not only the architect of the Arya Vaidya Sala but the renaissance leader of the revitalization movement of early twentieth century with its nucleus at Kottakkal. While alive, he dedicated his life to the cause of humanity and bequeathed, by his unique will, all that he inherited to posterity.

When the Arya Vaidya Sala completes hundred years of fruitful existence, the best tribute we can offer to the founder is the preservation of his personality for posterity. Ms Gita Krishnankutty, renowned for her literary pursuits, readily agreed to our request to prepare an authentic biography of the founder. With much pain she went through the annals of time and plunged deep to decipher his diaries to unravel the magnificence of his personality. We feel immensely indebted to her.

We are obliged to Penguin Books India for making this book available to the readers on the occasion of our centenary.

The life of P.S. Varier was a role model to his contemporaries; we hope it will be a source of inspiration to generations to come.

2 October 2001   Dr P.K. Warrier
Managing Trustee and Chief Physician
Kottakkal Arya Vaidya Sala

Prologue

The year 1886.

Vaidyam, a health care system which includes the learning and practice of the science of healing, was still being taught in the houses of the vaidyans according to the ancient gurukula system, in which a student stayed in the guru's house for as many years as it took him to complete what he had come to learn—from three or four to even ten, twelve years.

In the year 1886, there were many such sishyas in the illam or residence of Kuttanchery Vasudevan Mooss, a Namboodiri who belonged to one of the eight great reputed families of Ayurvedic physicians in Kerala, the ashtavaidyans, and a teacher who had trained many well-known vaidyans of the time. His illam was situated in a village called Ottupara in the interior of the erstwhile state of Cochin, near Vadakkanchery.

The illam was a modest one. It consisted of the main house—a traditional tiled structure, the nalukettu, built around a central sunken courtyard, the nadumuttam, with four wooden pillars at the corners; a gatehouse, also tiled, and a small kulappura, the building that overlooked the bathing tank belonging to the family. The tank itself has now shrunk to half its size, but the old kulappura still stands, amazingly untouched by time. The guru, Vasudevan Mooss, used to stay in a small room on the first floor and used the central hall adjacent to it as a classroom for his students. The students occupied the same building. Everyone ate in the main house, where the kitchen and women's quarters were situated.

The guru provided all the students who stayed in his house food, oil for their bath, and vaka powder or soap, whichever they used, to wash off the oil. The disciples brought their own clothes. They attended to their guru's personal needs from dawn to dusk not only in his own house but also on the occasions when they accompanied him on visits to the sick in other villages.

Among the students who came to take instruction from Kuttanchery Vasudevan Mooss in the year 1886 was a seventeen-year-old boy named Sankunni. With his long experience as a teacher, Mooss realized very quickly that this boy, serious by disposition, quick and eager to learn and the youngest of the group then residing at the illam, would be an excellent scholar and an exemplary disciple.

The daily routine at the illam was demanding and rigorous. The disciples had to rise at three. Their duties, which began at that hour of the day, included holding the lamp to light the guru's path when he went to perform his morning ablutions; heating water for him; laying out whatever he might want for his bath; gathering, preparing and arranging everything he needed for his lengthy puja rituals . . .

The older Namboodiris ate nothing until they had finished performing their long rituals of worship every morning. The first meal of the day at the illam was therefore often served only after noon. The male Namboodiris ate first, the Namboodiri women and children ate when the men had finished. Only then were people who belonged to other castes served. This meant that young Sankunni, who was not a Namboodiri, had his first meal only at two or three in the afternoon. He had come from a home where he had been used to eating a full meal at eight in the morning and initially, he must have found this change in routine hard to accept.

The instruction imparted to the young disciples by Vasudevan Mooss and Aryan Mooss, the other teacher in the household, was based on the study of Vagbhata's *Ashtangahridayam*, a text that all physicians in Kerala had to learn. This text describes the eight branches of treatment and is written in Sanskrit in the form of shlokas. The guru explained these verses to the disciples.

But the unique quality of the gurukula system was not simply the study of this text, nor the lucidity with which it was explained. It was the accumulation of everything a disciple imbibed by being with the guru, by accompanying him on his visits to sick patients, by closely observing, understanding and, above all, experiencing the diagnostic and therapeutic talents his guru exercised when he saw patients. Anubhavasiddhi, or the knowledge and powers earned through experience, was the acme of this school of learning.

One or two disciples always accompanied the guru on his visits to other villages. Besides carrying what they needed for themselves for the journey, the boys also carried on their heads the metal utensils the guru used for his puja, the clothes and oil he would need on the journey, his betel-leaf box and the granthams or palm-leaf manuscripts that he might have to consult. If the guru travelled in a bullock cart, it was generally driven by someone belonging to an inferior caste; if he travelled by palanquin, the same was true of the bearers. Since the rules of ritual purity were unrelenting in those days, the articles the disciples carried on their heads would have been polluted if they had been placed in the cart or palanquin. Physicians generally set out on such visits after their noon meal and, balancing heavy loads on their heads, the young boys ran behind the transport that carried their guru over rough cart tracks scorched by the sunlight, their bare feet burning.

One unforgettable day, an Ayurvedic physician who was a distant relative of Vasudevan Mooss came to visit him, accompanied by disciples overloaded with heavy sacks. After lunch, the visitor told Mooss that he wished to go on to another illam and that he would need one of his disciples to help carry his things. Vasudevan Mooss looked around to see which of them was in sight. Sensing what lay ahead, the older boys had discreetly disappeared and the only person he could see was his youngest and most loved disciple, Sankunni. Unwilling as he was to let the boy shoulder so heavy a burden, he was forced to ask him to go with the visitor. Sankunni came forward unhesitatingly, asking his guru for only one favour—permission to go home after he had reached the illam that was their destination, since his family lived nearby. The visitor's disciples, quick to snatch their chance, placed the heaviest of the three sacks, the one that contained innumerable bell-metal vessels, on the boy's head.

It was a hot summer's day and the sun blazed mercilessly overhead. Although they stopped now and then to rest their burdens on the stone platforms by the wayside, the journey, which took all of ten hours, seemed interminable. They arrived at the illam they were bound for only by nightfall. Exhausted, Sankunni slept there that night. When he reached his house the next day, he had a raging fever. Ordinary remedies did nothing to relieve it. The fever rose so high that he lost consciousness for a while.

At some point during the painful, delirium-racked days that followed, at a crucial moment during the illness that took such a heavy toll of him that it obliged him to stay home for a few months, interrupting his studies, a thought came to the boy, half-dream, half-vision: would it be possible some day for students like him, avid for learning, to pursue their studies without having to undergo such severe hardships and dedicate themselves single-mindedly to mastering Ayurveda?

It took all of three decades for that vision to take shape: in 1917, the young boy, by then known as P.S. Varier, Panniyinpally Sankunni Varier, established the Arya Vaidya Patasala, the first educational institution which taught Ayurveda in the town of Kozhikode in Malabar. The institution was to move a few years later to his home town, Kottakkal, where it stands today, a tribute to the perseverance and determination of its remarkable founder.

Kottakkal is a bustling little township today. Gleaming jewellery stores, colourful textile shops, stationery shops festooned with cheap plastic toys, furniture showrooms displaying wood finished in veneers ranging from pale white to rich maroon, jostle each other on the main road which is part of the National Highway Seventeen.

A narrow street veers at a sharp right angle to this main road and dips down a steep slope. Halfway along it is the small building in which P.S. Varier started the Arya Vaidya Sala, the first centre that sold ready-made Ayurvedic medicines in Kerala, a hundred years ago. The modest structure is dwarfed by the vast complex of office and factory buildings that surround it now. Across the street from it are the Ayurvedic Hospital and Research Centre that provides accommodation for in-patients who come to Kottakkal for long-term treatment. The Patasala established in 1917 has now become an Ayurveda College affiliated to Calicut University.

Vehicles belonging to the Arya Vaidya Sala ply up and down ceaselessly, carrying goods and passengers from the factory and Nursing Home in the heart of Kottakkal to the Ayurveda College, the Herb Garden, the Charitable Hospital, and to all the far-flung branches of the Arya Vaidya Sala in India.

'Do you remember your uncle, Sreedevi Cheriyamma?'

For eighty-seven-year-old Sreedevi Varasyar, P.S. Varier's niece and the oldest living member of the Panniyinpally family, known to everyone as Sreedevi Cheriyamma, the past and the present are inextricably woven together. The smile that starts in her bright eyes radiates to every contour of her face, to even the crisp curls of hair that frame it, as she answers: 'Of course. Do you know, all the children loved to play a game with him. They would run upstairs, stand on the veranda outside the big window opening into his rooms and call out to him. He would laugh loudly in answer and the next thing you saw was all of them diving, heads almost colliding, to catch the sudden shower of pastel-coloured peppermints that rained through the window, pale pink and green and creamy yellow, with letters of the English alphabet on them...'

Sreedevi Cheriyamma reaches out for a book on the table beside her. 'Shall I sing you the song he wrote in praise of Lord Vishvambhara?'

Her voice rises, true and clear:

> *Poornathrayiyil paripoornathma*
> *Shyanandapure seshashayan nee*
> *Vimalavaraha viharakshetre*
> *Visvambharanayvilaseedunnu*[1]

(You are the Complete One in Tripunithura, in the temple of Poorna Threyeeshan; You are Seshasayee, He Who Lies on the Serpent, in the temple at Thiruvananthapuram; in the temple of Panniyinpally [the house of the boar, Varaha], you are Vishvambharan.)

---

[1] A verse from the *Bhagavadkeshadipadam*, a long poem in praise of Vishnu, written by P.S. Varier.

1

The Beginnings

The Variers of Kerala are Ambalavasis, those who depend on the temple for their livelihood, and form the castes immediately below the Namboodiri Brahmins and above the Nairs. All Ambalavasis have rights and duties in the temple. It is the Variers who gather flowers and weave them into the garlands that adorn the deities. They wash all the things needed for the puja rituals in the temple, like the lamps and platters, as well as the utensils used in the temple kitchen. They sweep and clean the temple precincts, including the small sacrificial stones that the Namboodiri priests lay offerings upon during the sreebali procession. The Variers carry the koluvilakku, the oil lamp with a long handle, that is taken around the temple during this procession. In return for these services, they receive the cooked rice that has been offered to the gods, and land, if the temple is wealthy enough to give them some. The combination of their duties, which can be performed by both men and women of the Varier community, with whatever they receive from the temple in return, is known as a 'kazhakam'.

According to legend, the Variers or 'Parshwajans' were

brought to Kerala by Parasurama to be of assistance to the Brahmins whom he established in the region. However, groups called Variers are mentioned in Tamil stone inscriptions and are believed to have taken an active part in the village administration that took shape and developed under the Pallavas in Kanchipuram.[2] According to these inscriptions, Variers were those selected to form the committees that collected revenues. Inscriptions found in Uthiramerur in Tamil Nadu, speak of a Brahmin village in that area with a sophisticated system of village administration, in which the Variers, who were Brahmins themselves, worked on committees in charge of various aspects of living. There were panchavariams which dealt with five different kinds of revenue ('pancha' meaning five), ponvariams that were concerned with commerce in gold ('pon' meaning gold), thottavariams that looked after gardens that were public or royal property ('thottam' meaning garden), erivariams that were responsible for the water supply ('eri' meaning river) and so on. As temples gained in power and wealth, the koilvariam came into existence ('koil' meaning temple) and is mentioned in Chola inscriptions. Records of village administration in Kerala do not, however, mention Variers. The Variers of Kerala have always been associated with duties in the temple. N.V. Krishna Warrior thinks that when the Namboodiris became a powerful force in Kerala, they must have appointed some of their dependents to carry out duties that corresponded to the koilvariams in the temples; that these duties would have, over a period of time, become hereditary; that the name 'Varier' must have attached itself to the performance of such duties and eventually turned into the name of a caste. Raghava

---

[2] 'Variers and the Variam' (Varirayrum variyavum): N.V. Krishna Warrior, *The Golden Jubilee Souvenir* of the Arya Vaidya Sala, Kottakkal, 1954.

Varier and Rajan Gurukkal[3] speak of the Variers as holders of kazhakams in the Kerala temples and of inscriptions that indicate that tax-free lands were gifted to them in return for their services. These lands gradually became the wages for services rendered by a particular family, whose members took care to continue performing the tasks that fetched the wages, thereby making sure that the lands stayed in the family. Eventually, on the basis of the relationship they had with the temple and the lands they earned thereby, the Variers assumed a certain social status which, in turn, isolated them as a distinct caste.

However, the Variers of Kerala were not content to confine themselves to duties in the temple. In time, they became excellent astrologers, Sanskrit scholars, poets, dramatists, dedicated teachers and skilled vaidyans. They followed the marumakkathayam, the matrilineal system in which property is inherited through the women of the family and their children. Men had a right to own family property, but could not hand it down to their wives and children. The karanavan, the seniormost man in a matrilineal taravad or extended family, administered the properties and looked after family affairs; the other members, young and old, deferred to him.

P.S. Varier belonged to an ancient Varier family, the Panniyinpally taravad, whose original home was in Nanmanda, a small village in Malabar. The Panniyinpally Variers held a kazhakam in the local village temple. Over the years, the family fortunes flourished, the men pursued careers that took them beyond the temple precincts and the more successful among them were appointed to important and influential

[3]Raghava Varier and Rajan Gurukkal: *Kerala Charithram* (History of Keralam), Vallathol Vidyapeetam, 1991, p.147.

positions, like those of accountants and managers, at the court of the Raja of Kurumbranad, and in the army.

Towards the end of the eighteenth century, when Hyder Ali and after him, Tipu, invaded Malabar, many people fled southward in search of new ways of livelihood. Among them were the Panniyinpally Variers, who found their way to the state of Travancore, ruled then by Karthika Thirunal Rama Varma Raja. Two of them, Achutha Varier and Madhava Varier, were excellent artists. Their work found favour with the Raja of Travancore, who not only recognized and appreciated their talents, but also arranged for a kazhakam for them at the well-known temple in Ambalapuzha. The exquisite murals they executed on the walls of this temple, which included a 'Swayamvara Parvathy', attracted the attention of innumerable visitors to the area.

Many others from Malabar sought refuge at this period at Rama Varma Raja's court which was a famous centre for art and culture. Among them were two scholars who were to become generous patrons and friends of the Panninyinpally Varier family in later years. One of them was Manorama Thambatti, a princess belonging to the ruling family of Kozhikode, the Samoothiris, and an accomplished Sanskrit scholar. She had earned her name by mastering the *Manorama*, the annotated commentary on the *Siddhanta Kaumudi*, a grammar text, at the age of twelve. She spent almost twelve years with her husband and her two children in Travancore. The other person who befriended the Variers was the reputed Thambrakkal of the Azhvanchery Mana, a Namboodiri who was well-versed in the Vedas and an authority in all religious matters and rituals.

In 1799, the British annexed Karnataka and south Malabar and returned a portion of their land to the Samoothiris. The chieftains in the area had to accept British supremacy. Many people who had left Malabar and gone to south Kerala began to make their way back, among them Manorama Thambatti and the Azhvanchery Thambrakkal, both of whom went back around 1800.

Achutha Varier chose to stay on with his immediate family at Ambalapuzha, but the rest of the Panniyinpally family returned to Malabar under the guardianship of a senior member, Raghava Varier.

Anxious to re-establish the family fortunes in Malabar, Raghava Varier sought the help of the Azhvanchery Thambrakkal, who had been very friendly with the Panniyinpally family in Travancore. The Thambrakkal did not disappoint him. He arranged for the family to take over the kazhakam of a Subramania temple in south Malabar, in a village called Kottur, not far from the village of Kottakkal.

Meanwhile, Manorama Thambatti's brother, the third in the line of succession in the Samoothiri family, had taken up residence in the old Venkitta fort in the village of Kottakkal, where a branch of the royal family lived. He decided to renovate the ancient Shiva temple in the village, known locally as the Venkitta Thevar temple, and revive the pujas and festivals that had been interrupted when the family had moved away for a while and the temple had fallen into disuse. He accordingly had an elaborate purificatory ceremony performed. He then realized that there was a great deal of work to be done and the temple would require additional hands. When Manorama learnt that the Panniyinpally Variers, whom she had met in Travancore, were back in Malabar, she arranged for them to be given a kazhakam in the Venkitta Thevar temple.

A village that abounds with steep slopes, Kottakkal (meaning 'near a fort') derives its name from an ancient 'kotta', a fort, known as the Venkitta Kotta, situated near the Shiva temple. The village was originally a wilderness until the Samoothiri took it over in the early eighteenth century and established a kovilakam, a palace, there. Following this, the village began to grow and develop. When Tipu captured this region, he widened the roads and renovated the fort.

Once Manorama Thambatti and the other members of her family came back from Travancore, the residents of the kizhakke kovilakam or eastern palace grew in numbers and became a strong force in the village of Kottakkal. Many people came from outside Kottakkal seeking the patronage of the palace or work of some kind in the vicinity and the members of the royal family were generous with help. The thampuran who was the head of the palace from 1859 to 1878 did much to improve the quality of life in Kottakkal. He built a marketplace and brought Muslim traders from Parappanangadi to do business in Kottakkal. He constructed a gopuram for the temple and built its outer walls.

The Venkitta Thevar temple which still stands today, is believed to be well over five hundred years old. It has some of the most exquisite murals that can be seen in Kerala on the walls of the sreekovil, the sanctuary, said to be the work of an artist named Edayattu Sankaran Nair.

Another Varier clan, the Manalil Thrikkovil family, who had, like the Panniyinpally Variers, moved briefly to Travancore and returned later to Malabar had also been given a kazhakam in the Subramania temple at Kottur. The Panniyinpally Variers were therefore able to leave the Kottur temple in their charge and shift to Kottakkal to take up their new duties under the guardianship of Raghava Varier. They first stayed in a small house east of the kovilakam. In 1825, when the royal family decided to put up buildings that would extend over the land the Variers occupied, Raghava Varier moved south of the temple and built a small house that came to be known as the southern variam.

The matrilineal joint family of Kerala comprises the male head of the family, the seniormost in age, his sisters and their children. Raghava Varier's family consisted of two nephews,

Govinda Varier and Anantha Varier, two nieces, Parvathy Varasyar and Ittichiri Varasyar—the women in Varier families are known as Varasyars—and the children of these nephews and nieces.

Govinda Varier was accomplished in astrology and vaidyam. He eventually became a disciple of one of the most reputed Namboodiri vaidyans of the time, Pulamanthole Mooss, and moved to his illam.

After spending a few years in Kottakkal, Anantha Varier decided to find out what had happened to the original home of the Panniyinpally Variers in Nanmanda. He discovered that their property now belonged to a Namboodiri named the Panniyinpally Bhattadiripad, who had taken over the deserted Panniyinpally house. Anantha Varier could find no trace of the family temple or of the bathing tanks adjacent to it.

He was initially disheartened, but his journey did not prove entirely fruitless. The people of the village remembered his family, welcomed him warmly, extended all the help he needed to set up house and arranged a kazhakam for him in the Nanmanda temple. He therefore settled down in Nanmanda and soon married a woman from one of the Varier families there.

What he did not know was that the senior members of his family who had left the village and gone to Travancore had secretly removed their household deity from the temple and hidden it in the bathing tank, fearing it might be desecrated in their absence.

The Bhattadiripad who had taken over the old Panniyinpally family house was somehow not able to live in it peacefully. Beset by innumerable domestic worries all the time, he finally decided to arrange for astrologers to do a prasnam, a ritual which would help them assess his situation and find a remedy for it. The astrologers would throw cowries into formations that would determine the precise position of the planets and then suggest ways to ward off their evil effects. One of the discoveries the astrologers made in this way was that the old idol still lay hidden at the spot where the temple tank had been. It was eventually found and taken out and a new temple was built to consecrate it.

To this day, the Variers of the Panniyinpally family who live in Kottakkal visit Nanmanda to offer worship to their ancient household deity.

Raghava Varier's nieces Parvathy Varasyar and Ittichiri Varasyar, who stayed with him at Kottakkal, had eight children between them: all sons with one exception.

Ittichiri Varasyar had four sons, Shoolapani, Sankaran, Madhavan and Achuthan. Three of them learned vaidyam from the most reputed Ayurvedic physicians of the period. Shoolapani went to Vayaskara Mooss, Sankaran to Pulamanthole Mooss and Madhavan to Kuttanchery Mooss. Shoolapani died young, but the other two physicians earned great reputations in their field. Sankaran became the family physician at the eastern kovilakam, and his professional fame spread throughout the region. Madhavan was the family physician at the western kovilakam, the palace at Kozhikode. Disciples from within the palace and outside flocked to him to learn vaidyam. Achuthan, the youngest of the four, became the personal advisor to Manorama Thambatti's son, Shaktan Thampuran.

Parvathy Varasyar also had four children, three sons and a daughter: Raman, Bharathan, Lakshmi and Easwaran. Inheriting his great-uncle Raghava Varier's mantle, Raman rose to the position of manager of the Cherukunnu temple, which belonged to the royal family. Bharatha Varier, who distinguished himself in astrology, became the legal manager of the senior thamburatti at the palace. The youngest child, Easwaran, started life as an earnest and gifted scholar, but became deranged later in life.

Lakshmi, Parvathy Varasyar's daughter, was the only hope the Panniyinpally family now had of survival. Since the Variers follow the matrilineal line of inheritance, it was on Lakshmi that the continuance of the line depended.

Lakshmi Varasyar, also known as Kunji, was married to Krishna Varier of the Deshamangalam family. Hereditarily, the men of the Deshamangalam family were great scholars and many of them were teachers in the Samoothiri household.

Three children were born of this union: Krishnan, known as Kuttikrishnan, was born in 1831; Parvathy, known as Kunjukutty, in 1839 and Ittichiri, known as Kutty, in 1841.

Kuttikrishnan became a distinguished Sanskrit scholar and also learned vaidyam. Both the sisters were excellent scholars of Sanskrit as well. In addition they became accomplished musicians. It was a period when few women were expert in music, especially in Malabar. Both sisters were therefore greatly sought after as teachers of music and acquired many students, including the women of the kovilakam.

Kunjukutty was married to Marayamangalathu Mangulangara Rama Varier. He was then the manager of the eastern palace in Kottakkal and stayed at the palace. Kutty, the other sister, was first married to her father's nephew, Deshamangalam Shekhara Varier. Later, when the family moved to their house in Mangulangara, she was married to a wealthy landlord named Cherukulapurathu Namboodiri. However, even after many years of marriage, neither sister had children. This became a source of deep anxiety for the family—if they remained childless, the Panniyinpally line would die out. Since, by this time, there were no more women belonging to the Panniyinpally family in those branches that had settled in Ambalapuzha and Nanmanda, they were already doomed to extinction. Would the same fate befall the branch at Kottakkal? Worry haunted them, gave their minds no rest. The family performed many charitable acts and made generous donations and offerings to various temples. When these bore no results, they thought they would turn to astrology and have a prasnam conducted. Meanwhile, their neighbours and well-wishers in the village were concerned for them. The Variers' home was situated to the right of the deity in the Venkitta Thevar temple: this was inauspicious, the women of the family would not be able to bear children. The villagers spoke of others living in that area who had been similarly affected in this way.

The elders in the family thought it wise to accept the truth of what they said and decided to move from Kottakkal.

Since Kunjukutty's husband, Rama Varier, belonged to Mangulangara, he thought he would build a house there for his wife's family to live in. He already had a kazhakam in the local temple. The Panniyinpally family obtained one in the same temple for themselves since it was not considered fitting for Variers not to have a kazhakam.

The house that was being constructed in Mangulangara was to be called the eastern variam. However, in 1864, before the house was ready, Lakshmi Varasyar died suddenly. An infinitely gentle person in looks and manner, she had assumed charge of household affairs from the age of ten or twelve and managed them with quiet efficiency. She had not had much education, but had always been a remarkably capable wife and mother. Her death left the whole family feeling orphaned.

The construction of the new variam was expedited and the move from Kottakkal to Mangulangara was made the same year.

Both Kunjukutty and Kutty had been married before they came of age, according to the custom in those days—Kunjukutty had, in fact, been only twelve years old. Their childlessness continued to be a source of deep anxiety. It was decided to consult an astrologer in Pazhoor, a well-known man who had a reputation for never making a mistake. He conducted a prasnam and asked the family to perform a number of pujas in the temple, make various offerings and chant certain prayers. His instructions were carried out faithfully.

The gods relented: before long, Kutty, the younger sister, found herself pregnant. In 1867, she gave birth to a daughter who was named Lakshmi, after her late grandmother.

There was great rejoicing in the family. The birth of a daughter was especially significant, for it meant that the family line would continue and that the ominous threat of extinction no longer existed. Kunjukutty, the older sister, whose attachment to her younger sister was extremely strong and whose sense of family was deep and loyal, was neither disappointed nor envious because she herself had not conceived. Her sister's daughter would perpetuate the Panniyinpally taravad and this mattered far more to her than her own childlessness.

Kunjukutty Varasyar was a woman of exceptional qualities. Besides being accomplished in literature and music, she had taken over the management of the household after her mother's death, at the age of twenty-five, and learned to run it with great efficiency. Intelligent and resourceful, she had a phenomenal memory. The villagers often pawned their jewels and borrowed money from her. It was said that she never kept accounts of these transactions and that she stored every detail concerning them, even the most minute one, in her memory. She knew the date on which each person had borrowed money from her, how much she had lent and what sum they owed her at any moment, inclusive of interest.

There is a wonderful legend in the family of how the temple authorities once mislaid the palm leaf scrolls containing the details of the long lists of rituals that had to be performed at the annual festival. Kunjukutty Varasyar not only recited the lists to the temple officials from memory, she dispatched the abashed officials with a stern warning to write the details down at once, put them away safely and not mislay them and ask her to repeat everything all over again! The people of Kottakkal sought her advice in times of trouble. It was said that Manorama Thambatti's son, Shaktan Thampuran, often sent envoys to her from the kovilakam to seek her opinion on local problems.

Her husband, Mangulangara Rama Varier, was a deeply religious man, straightforward and meticulous in all his dealings. While most people who had experienced his kindness and generosity thought highly of him, those who had been unfortunate enough to fall out with him feared his integrity and outspokenness.

The arrival of Kutty Varasyar's daughter had rekindled the hope that the Panniyinpally line would go on, but a new misgiving began to torment the family. Ittichiri Varasyar's sons, Sankara Varier and Madhava Varier, had established a reputation as eminent vaidyans. Who would inherit their professional acumen and carry on this tradition? When the astrologer at Pazhoor performed a prasnam, he had predicted that Kunjukutty would have a son who would fulfil his parent's hopes and grow up to be the heir who would perform their funeral rites. But Kunjukutty was now nearly thirty years old. Would the prediction come true? Although the family continued to pray and make offerings to the gods, their hopes began to dwindle.

Krishna Varier did not enjoy the happiness of having become a grandfather for long. He died soon after his granddaughter Lakshmi was born.

2

Birth and Childhood

The family's continued prayers were finally answered: Kunjukutty Varasyar became pregnant. Bharatha Varier, the seniormost in the Panniyinpally family now, took up residence in Mangulangara in order to be present at the childbirth. Kunjukutty was not young anymore and they were all worried. What if something went wrong? If the astrologer's prediction proved true, there was hope that this child would also inherit the excellent reputation Sankara Varier and Madhava Varier had established in the field of vaidyam.

On 16 March 1869 Kunjukutty Varasyar gave birth to a boy. The child's birth star was Ashwini.

The happy news spread rapidly through the village and visitors flocked to the house to have a look at the baby. He was unusually big and many visitors remarked that there was more than enough to see of the long-awaited child! Kunjukutty Varasyar herself was delighted, but her loyalty to the family was so deep that she declared that her joy at having had a son was in no way comparable to the greater happiness she had experienced when her younger sister gave birth to the daughter who would carry their line forward; she described it as a

complete and extraordinary happiness, the like of which she
was certain she would never experience again.

Sankara Varier, who had been the physician at the Kottakkal
palace, had died a few months before Kunjukutty Varasyar had
her baby. The child was therefore named Sankaran after his
great-uncle. He was called Sankunni for short, and sometimes,
members of the family called him Kuttan.

Kunjukutty did not have any more children. Kutty had a
second daughter, Madhavi, in 1872, a son, Krishnan
(Kunjukuttan) in 1877 and a third daughter, Parvathy in 1884.

Sankunni's vidyarambham, the ceremony conducted to
initiate him into writing on Vijayadashami day, the last day of
the nine-day Navarathri festival, took place before he was four
years old. His uncle, Kuttikrishna Varier, helped him to write
his letters and became his first teacher.

Not long after this, however, this uncle fell ill. Sankunni's
mother therefore began to spend long periods of time at
Kottakkal to take care of her brother. At these times, her
younger sister Kutty and both the children, Lakshmi and
Sankunni, would accompany her. And so a great part of
Sankunni's childhood was spent in Kottakkal.

Whenever he was at Kottakkal, the people of the village
would tease the little boy who bore his vaidyan great-uncle's
name. Hey Uncle Sankunni, they would call out, I have a
headache, a stomach ache. Can you suggest some medicine to
cure it? Sankunni would prescribe a remedy with perfect
seriousness: grind some muthanga grass, he would reply, and
smear its paste on your forehead; or, roast and powder dried
ginger, mix it in buttermilk and drink it . . .

Circumstances forced Sankunni anyway into a seriousness
and sense of responsibility beyond his years. In 1874, when he
was five years old, his great-uncle, Rama Varier, Parvathy
Varasyar's eldest son, died. Rama Varier's younger brother,
Easwara Varier, died four months later.

It was the custom in those days for a nephew of the deceased person to observe a period of mourning called deeksha, that lasted a full year. Fasting once a day, he had to grow a beard, remain celibate and perform the rites for the dead every day over the whole year. It fell to Kuttikrishna Varier, Sankunni's uncle, to perform these rites for his two uncles. But he was himself a feeble person, already in ill health. He died three months after Easwara Varier passed away. The only senior member now left was Parvathy Varasyar's second son, Bharatha Varier. He was far too old and weak to perform the deeksha rituals. Not to have the rituals performed was unthinkable, but who was to do them?

The next in line was five-year-old Sankunni. The elders pondered over the weighty question and finally decided that the child had to take on this grim responsibility, young as he was.

Kunjukutty Varasyar and Sankunni had to therefore stay in Kottakkal so that the boy could perform the rites. The discipline of that year was severe: Sankunni had to get up very early in the morning, have a dip in the tank and perform the rituals in dripping wet clothes. He had to eat extremely simple food and deny himself all the small, carefree pleasures of childhood. His mother, although she loved him deeply—her only child—always expected perfection from him. That year's exacting routine taught him a discipline which was to stand him in good stead all his life.

Sankunni's seven-year-old cousin, Lakshmi, Kutty Varasyar's daughter, also moved to Kottakkal with them. She stayed with her Valiamma for the next twelve years and became the sibling Sankunni had never had. The children grew deeply attached to each other, a bond that lasted throughout their lives.

The daily rituals for the deeksha period were performed at Kottakkal but for the final rites, which required the participation of many people, they moved briefly to Mangulangara.

When the period of mourning was over, Kunjukutty Varasyar stayed on at Kottakkal. Sankunni began his real education with Killimangalam (or Ikkandath) Krishna Varier, who was then living at the palace in Kottakkal. He studied Sanskrit kavyam to begin with.

Other teachers, like his own uncle Bharatha Varier, Chunakkara Kochukrishna Varier and Ananthanarayana Iyer, a well-known astrologer, also took classes for Sankunni from time to time.

Kaikulangara Rama Varier, a great scholar of the period and the author of excellent commentaries on many Sanskrit texts, came to stay at the kovilakam for some time and taught the young boy for a while. He inspired him with a love for poetry and urged him to try his hand at writing verse. Sankunni attempted his first sloka under his tutelage:

Vande narayanam devam nutanambudamechakam
Shankachakragadapadma-dharam garudavahanam

(I praise Him, Narayanan, the God who has the black hue of nascent clouds, who bears the conch, discus, club and lotus in His hands, who has Garuda as His vehicle.)

Killimangalam Krishna Varier first held his classes in the outhouse of the temple, then shifted them to the kovilakam after six months. In later years Sankunni used to recall with great pleasure the bonds he forged with the young boys who studied with him at this time. Many members of the family recalled him talking about one of these boys, Ramakrishna Iyer, who hated to study. Every day, his father used to carry him into class, kicking and protesting, and leave him with the guru. But the boy would slip out at the first chance he got and play truant. One day, Sankunni thought he too would play truant and find out how it felt to stay away from class. So he hid all day in the building overlooking the bathing tank, going home briefly only to have lunch. He was deeply disappointed:

time hung heavy on his idle hands and he was very bored, with nothing to do except gaze at the fishes darting through the water! He never tried the experiment again.

It was a period of time when parents who could afford it were very anxious to teach their children English and Sankunni himself was quite eager to learn the language. But his parents wanted their son to master Sanskrit before he started a study of vaidyam and would not hear of him learning English.

Sankunni's teacher, Krishna Varier, had to leave very suddenly for his village and his next teacher was Deshamangalam Kunjikrishna Varier, who was also his cousin Lakshmi's husband.

Sankunni's life as a student was interrupted again when Bharatha Varier, the last of his great-uncles, died in 1881. Barely twelve years old, Sankunni once again found himself the seniormost male member of his family. Since Bharatha Varier had been living in the kovilakam for many years, looking after its affairs as their manager, the palace authorities provided Sankunni with the funds to conduct the year-long deeksha rituals for him.

At the end of that year, when the deeksha was over, Sankunni requested the kovilakam to continue giving him funds, but the thampuran who was in charge of the finances refused to do so. He told the boy that he would hover around the kovilakam all his life if they kept giving him money and never learn vaidyam. This must have seemed a harsh decision to the young boy, but at this crucial juncture, it served to propel him into a career of study that was to last for many years and shape his destiny. He was to realize later that it was the best advice he could have received at that moment in his life.

However, before he applied himself to the study of vaidyam, he had to first complete his study of Sanskrit.

How had proficiency in the Sanskrit language become an integral part of the study of vaidyam?

There are parallel streams in the growth and development of the health care systems in Kerala and obviously, not all of them insisted on a thorough knowledge of Sanskrit. Clearly, many special features of vaidyam in Kerala, the knowledge of the uses of certain drugs and herbs native to the region and of methods of treatment used only in Kerala must have existed before the arrival of Sanskrit. The medicinal properties of the tender coconut, for instance, are recognized only in Kerala. Ancient Ayurvedic texts also acknowledge the use of many parts of the coconut in the manufacture of medicines. Modes of treatment like dhara (a procedure in which liquids are made to flow over, more or less to irrigate, the head or the body), navara kizhi (the application of heated poultices filled with a variety of rice known as navara, the ideal grain being one called shashtikam, grown over sixty days), pizhichil and uzhichil (dipping a piece of cloth in heated oil and applying it on the body, gently stroking it all the while) are practices special to Kerala and must certainly have existed well before the arrival of the Sanskrit language.

Nor was vaidyam in Kerala necessarily the exclusive domain of the Brahmins. There have been and still are many Ezhava practitioners of vaidyam who have learnt Sanskrit and who add the title 'vaidyan' to their names. Sree Narayana Guru, the spiritual leader of the Ezhava community, belonged to a family of vaidyans and was one himself.

Among many of the so-called lower castes in Kerala, secret knowledge about certain methods of treatment, about the properties and powers of certain drugs, were handed down from father to son. The women of the washerman community, for instance, were traditionally skilled in midwifery, while the men were excellent paediatricians. Kurups, another caste, were excellent at the different types of massage used for pizhichil and uzhichil courses of treatment. There were entire families who were expert in specific branches like paediatrics, eye diseases or treatment administered to victims of poisoning. Similarly, there were families who specialized in the use of particular drugs or herbs for wounds. As in all ancient civilizations, the practice of vaidyam in Kerala was associated with witchcraft and sorcery.

Around the sixth century, the Namboodiri Brahmins began to dominate the society of Kerala. The power they wielded was based on their priestly right to conduct sacrificial rituals, yagas. Because they were well-versed in the Vedas, Sanskrit, the language of the Vedas, grew in importance. The lands that lay around the temples were donated to the Namboodiris, and they gradually became land-holders in addition to being priests. Temples became centres for the study of Sanskrit. They also acquired a reputation for the treatment of specific diseases: like the Kodungalloor temple for smallpox and the Chottanikkara temple for mental instability.

As this upper-caste section of society grew stronger, wealthy and influential Namboodiri families began to feel a need for physicians from their own caste. They began to have at least one member in each family trained in vaidyam. Once established, these Namboodiri vaidyans began to treat princes and nobles, which meant they could amass more wealth and power.

The ashtavaidyans who eventually became known as great scholars and teachers of vaidyam in Kerala are all Namboodiris. The prefix 'ashta' denotes eight. In addition, it is also believed that it is because they mastered the *Ashtangahridayam*, Vagbhata Acharya's great treatise on Ayurveda, that these physicians came to be known as ashtavaidyans.[4] The eight families of ashtavaidyans who earned a reputation for excellence during this period and still retain it are: Pulamanthole, Alathiyoor,

---

[4] N.V.Krishnankutty Warrior: *Ayurveda Charithram* (History of Ayurveda), Arya Vaidya Sala, Kottakkal, 1980.

Kuttanchery, Thrissur Thaykkat, Vayaskara, Chirattaman, Vellote and Karthol. Of these, the Alathiyoor and Karthol families are known as Nambi, all the others are known as Mooss. There were particular Namboodiri families who specialized in witchcraft and performed rites of exorcism, others acquired great skill in treating victims bitten by snakes.

The Namboodiri Ayurvedic physicians in Kerala were always open to different trends in vaidyam. Vagbhata's works are acknowledged as a fundamental part of the study of Ayurveda in Kerala although he is a Buddhist. Indu, one of the finest exponents of Vagbhata's text, is believed to be from Kerala. However, vaidyam was always considered a slightly inferior profession by those Namboodiris who were scholars of the Vedas.

Since the texts the Namboodiri teachers taught were originally written in Sanskrit, a mastery over the language became imperative for students who wanted to learn vaidyam from them.

Sankunni therefore applied himself to the study of Sanskrit under Kunjikrishna Varier. He first did poetry, then logic and grammar.

In 1885, Kunjikrishna Varier fell ill and died. Sankunni was now sixteen. He had acquired the proficiency he needed in Sanskrit and was ready to embark on the study of vaidyam.

3

The Life of a Student

In 1885, Sankunni began to study the fundamental chapters in vaidyam with Konath Achutha Varier, the resident vaidyan at the kovilakam in Kottakkal and a disciple of Kuttanchery Mooss. He completed the study of yogam (the formulations of compounds of drugs), chikitsakramam (therapeutic routines including the administration of medicines) and gunapatam (the pharmaceutical properties of drugs and materials) with this teacher.

He now had to go to an ashtavaidyan, enrol as a disciple and start his gurukulavasam as a resident in the guru's house. Sankunni decided to go to Kuttanchery Vasudevan Mooss, who was reputed to be one of the best teachers at that period and was the guru of many well-known physicians of the time.

In 1886, Sankunni embarked on what was to prove a memorable and deeply rewarding phase of his life as one of the disciples in the illam of Vasudevan Mooss.

The little village of Ottupara near Vadakkanchery is now only a straggle of houses, partly old and partly new, lying off the main road that winds through it. In the 1880s, Mooss's illam must have been the pivot of the village, its pulsating heart, with the young boys who were his disciples hurrying to and fro as they attended to their varied duties, and streams of sick people coming to the renowned physician for advice and treatment from many parts of Kerala.

The ancient Dhanvanthari family temple still stands, barely touched by the passage of time. Vasudevan Mooss's grandfather or great-grandfather, it is not quite certain who built it. He used to walk five miles every morning to Nelluvaya to worship Dhanvanthari, the god of healing, the deity of the temple there, until he grew too old and weak for this daily excursion. Reluctant to discontinue a practice that had become part of his life, he obtained permission to instal another form of the idol of Nelluvaya in a temple he built in his own illam compound. There is a small stone statue of Dhanvanthari in the central shrine, a Ganapathy to the side and a Shiva shrine. All the shrines and the corridors connecting them have very low tiled roofs. Vasudevan Mooss's young students must certainly have hit their heads against them time and again as they hurried in and out at the hours of worship! Adjacent to the temple is a vast bathing tank. The solid walls demarcating the different bathing ghats and the steps that lead down to the water are of gleaming black granite.

The old illam has been demolished, so has the gatehouse. But the little two-storeyed building overlooking the bathing tank is intact and so is the tank itself, though it has obviously shrunk in size with time. Vasudevan Mooss and his students stayed in this building. The guru slept in a small room upstairs and taught his students in the central hall adjoining it. Steps lead down to the tank from the ground floor of the little building. Namboodiris and students from the Ambalavasi and Nair communities stayed in this house and ate their meals at the illam.

The instruction imparted by the guru was based mainly on

Vagbhata's *Ashtangahridayam* and the explication of the verses it contained. This treatise deals with eight branches of treatment and codifies information with regard to each branch. They are: kaya chikitsa or treatment of the body; shalya chikitsa or surgery; bala chikitsa or the treatment of children, including the newborn; bhoothavidya or the treatment of mental diseases or diseases induced by the evil effects of the planets; oordhvanga chikitsa, which is the treatment of everything that is situated above the Adam's apple; agatha tantram which includes the treatment for bites, stings and internally imbibed poisons; rasayana chikitsa which deals with rejuvenation and geriatric disorders and vajeekaranam, which is the treatment of diseases of the reproductory organs. The method of instruction varied with each guru and depended to a great extent on the individual student's grasp of Sanskrit and his ability to memorize the texts and recognize whatever the guru quoted from them.

While examining a patient and deciding on the course of treatment he should prescribe, the guru would quote a verse from the chapter where the kind of symptoms the patient had were described and then cite the yogam, the specific formulation used to process the medicine for those symptoms. The student was expected to situate the verse in the chapter it belonged to, and be able to make up the medicine according to the formulation mentioned in it. A strict guru would often refrain from repeating the verse, if his student had not been quick enough to grasp it. Periods of study varied and so did their intensity: often, students could learn far more from a practical session, watching their guru examine, diagnose and prescribe than from hours of learning a text by rote. Alertness, sharp observation, an ability to consistently relate verses from the ancient texts to practical modes of application: these were the qualities that a gurukula disciple had to train himself to develop.

The disciples attended to their guru's needs from the time

they woke up at dawn to when the guru retired to sleep at night. Most of the lazier boys quickly learnt how to evade the more difficult tasks, leaving them to the younger ones to perform. Being the youngest of the group at the Kuttanchery illam at that time, Sankunni often found himself carrying out tasks that his seniors had cleverly escaped from. But he was a dedicated disciple and, far from protesting, he enjoyed this privilege since it gave him greater opportunities to be with his guru, to observe and learn from him.

The mother of Aryan Mooss, the other teacher in the illam, was in charge of household affairs. She grew very fond of Sankunni. She particularly appreciated the meticulous manner in which he cleaned the spot where he ate every day. Picking up any rice grains that had scattered, he would sprinkle the whole area with water, mop it and smear it afresh with cowdung paste to make it ritually pure. For Sankunni, this was not a chore at all. His mother had trained him from the time he was a child to assist in keeping the temple premises clean. Traditionally, in the Kottakkal Venkitta Thevar temple, only men performed the cleaning tasks. In addition, Variers themselves always cooked the food they ate at the weddings and funerals of their own people. All those who attended these functions were expected to help with the cooking and serving and Sankunni was used to working hard on such occasions.

Aryan Mooss's mother grew so partial to young Sankunni that she would keep aside sweets and delicacies for him. If she realised a meal was going to be served unusually late because some ritual was likely to be unduly prolonged, she would send for him and give him something left over from the previous day so that he would not go hungry.

One or two disciples always accompanied the guru when he went to visit patients in other villages. For Sankunni, these journeys were often a great delight for another reason. When travelling by bullock-cart, his guru would ask the cart driver to get down and walk and tell Sankunni to take the reins. The boy would feel tremendously exhilarated as he arranged the sack he was carrying in the cart, jumped in and urged the animals forward and they picked up speed in obedience to his commands.

When Vasudevan Mooss was on a visit to a patient, he took special care to see that Sankunni's meals were not inordinately delayed. As soon as he finished eating, he would insist that Sankunni be served. The hosts never dared to object since he had a reputation for being hot-tempered and they had all heard of instances where Mooss had departed angrily with his attendants if he felt his instructions had not been obeyed.

Whenever Vasudevan Mooss went on a visit, people would flock to consult him from all over the neighbourhood, his reputation as an efficient physician being close to a legend. However, once he had examined the principal patient he had been summoned to see, Mooss would tell his hosts, 'I have to teach Sankunni now,' and conduct a class for the boy before he examined the others. This was an unusual and valuable concession, for gurus did not always maintain a regular teaching schedule while travelling and students had to rely completely on what they learnt through observation during these periods.

The vaidyan who arrived on a visit on the fateful day when Sankunni fell ill and his studies were disrupted had acquired a reputation for travelling with far more than he really needed and his disciples particularly dreaded the large collection of bell-metal vessels used for puja rituals that he always insisted on taking along everywhere. This was why all Sankunni's companions made themselves scarce as soon as the noon meal was over, for they were sure the visitor would ask their guru to send one of them along to carry his sacks. Sankunni was the only one who remained near his guru. He had never been afraid of hard work or of physical strain of any kind, and he always valued any opportunity he found to serve his guru.

That particular day, however, when it fell to him to carry the visitor's sack of bell-metal vessels, he might have already been ill when he started on the journey, for the strain of it proved too much for him.

Sankunni made his way to Mangulangara the day after he arrived at the illam Vasudevan Mooss's relative had been bound for. His parents were at Kottakkal, but Kutty Varasyar, his Cheriyamma, was at Mangulangara. When Sankunni fell ill and she found that the boys's fever would not respond to any remedy, Kutty Varasyar grew very anxious and sent for his father, who immediately came from Kottakkal. His mother, however, stayed back and spent those days in prayer, confident that her younger sister would care for Sankunni as if he were her own son.

Sankunni's illness lasted twenty-two days and took a heavy toll of him, leaving him too weak and tired to go back to Kuttanchery and resume his routine there. Anxious not to lose touch with his studies, he asked Vasudevan Mooss for permission to go back to Achutha Varier, his first teacher at the kovilakam and continued studying with him for some time.

He returned to Vasudevan Mooss after six months, by which time he had recovered. During the period that followed, until he finished his studies, the unexpressed longing he had experienced during his illness for a system of education that combined the best in the gurukulam method of study with an organized routine, must have lain dormant in his mind. But it is certain that he kept this thought completely under control through the years he spent at Vasudevan Mooss's illam, never allowing it to disturb the rhythm of his life as a dedicated disciple or interfere in any way with his concentration on his studies or with his devotion to his teacher.

In 1890, he finished his studies with his guru. He spent the whole of the following year in prayer and fasting at the Dhanvanthari temple in Nelluvaya, staying in a variam nearby.

During this period he mastered the last two sections of the *Ashtangahridayam* on his own: vikriti (the study of the premonitory symptoms of death) and doothu (the signs apparent in the messenger who brings news of a patient's illness). Once again, this must have been a period of intense discipline, self-imposed this time and without even the trivial distractions that companions of his age would have offered. Did the thought ever cross his mind as he prayed and studied in the temple that he would soon dedicate his life to evolving a system of learning that was going to be radically different from what he himself had been so committed to?

On Vijayadashami day in 1891, he offered his gurudakshina, the gift the student makes to the guru when he departs after a course of study, to his teachers at the Kuttanchery illam and left for Kottakkal. What did the disciple who had finished a course charted by the rules of gurukulavasam take with him when he went away into a new life? There had been no formal examination; Sankunni carried away no diploma, no medals or trophies. What he took with him was far more precious: a blessing whose radiance had touched his mind and heart and would mould his every future thought; the deep and warm affection of a teacher for a student who had fulfilled his promise; the invaluable knowledge and experience he had garnered by constantly watching his guru exercise his capacities as a physician. Sankunni was filled with gratitude.

The difficult moments no longer seemed relevant—the times he had walked long distances in the hot sun and then bathed in tanks in which the water was polluted; the frequent baths he had been obliged to have, once again in the dirty water of strange tanks, because ritual purity required it; the inability to have regular oil baths because he did not have enough time for them. All these had actually combined to aggravate an irritation in his eyes, the initial symptoms of an eye ailment that was to grow worse in later years. When it first

began, he had found that his congested eyes cleared and the
discomfort he felt when he faced the glare of sunlight improved
as soon as he had an oil bath. However, the rare oil baths he
could manage had gradually ceased to have a beneficial effect
on these symptoms. But he knew all this was negligible in the
light of what he had learnt at his guru's feet.

Nor had Sankunni's days at the Kuttanchery illam been
lacking in the lighter and more enjoyable aspects of life. He
had made many friends of his age, the closest of them being
Thaykatt Narayanan Mooss, a lively and amusing companion.
Once the guru finished his night meal and retired to sleep, the
boys used to laugh and joke with one another and play
harmless pranks. Sankunni had participated in all this
wholeheartedly and taken great pleasure in sharing in the fun
and amusement of his companions.

On his way back to Kottakkal, ready to start life as a
vaidyan, Sankunni must surely have wondered what the future
held for him and allowed his thoughts to mould, tentatively,
its still uncertain shape.

4

The Restless Years

As soon as he returned to Kottakkal, Sankunni began to see a few patients and prescribe treatment for their ailments. But he quickly realized that he would never be content to limit himself to remaining an ordinary village physician. He was restless for other kinds of knowledge, particularly in the area of western medicine (English vaidyam as it was known then, since it was the British who taught and practised it in India), which was by then slowly gaining popularity. There had been nothing so far in his background or his experience to awaken an ambition of this kind. This curiosity, this determination to explore avenues of knowledge that were not, strictly speaking, directly accessible to a young man in his position were to guide him into many uncharted territories and prove the driving forces of his life.

For the moment, however, the first obstacle he had to surmount was his ignorance of the English language, which he had wanted to learn from the time he was a child and never been able to. Attending school with very young children was unthinkable at his age and he did not have the means to go away from Kottakkal to find a teacher.

He discovered to his relief that there were members of the royal family at the eastern kovilakam who knew English and would teach him. So he started to learn the language with Kuttiettan Thampuran, an active worker in the Kerala Mahajana Sabha, who was willing to give up his afternoon siesta every day to teach him. Before long, a school was started on the kovilakam premises to teach English to whoever wanted to learn and Sankunni enrolled there.

Kutti Anujan Thampuran, one of the members of the royal family, taught in this school. Generous and kind-hearted, he had great concern for his students and, besides teaching English, he offered them much valuable advice during his classes on how to confront life. Sankunni reached the Lower Secondary School level of English in a year's time. He did not appear for the examination, however, because constant study and reading had aggravated his eye problem. He tried various kinds of treatment but they were ineffective, and the fact that he read long hours only served to make his condition worse.

Meanwhile, he had been continuing to see patients, some of whom came to his house and some of whom he visited in their homes. While he had always been an earnest and dedicated student of Ayurveda, ways and means to modify the manner in which it was practised constantly occupied his thoughts from the time he began his life as a vaidyan. Even while dealing with his first patients, he wished he could somehow process the medicines he prescribed for them himself and make it easy for them to start their treatment at once.

Ayurvedic medicines were not at all easy to procure. After making a diagnosis, physicians of the time wrote their prescriptions on palm leaf scrolls. The patients and their relatives had to first arrange for the ingredients for the prescription to be collected. They were of two kinds: those that could be bought in a shop and raw ingredients like roots, leaves and herbs that had to be plucked from the spot where they grew by people who had the knowledge and experience necessary to identify them. Once the ingredients were ready, the medicine had to be processed according to the proportions and methods of the formulation mentioned in the prescription. Special care had to be taken to mix it or heat it over a fire to the required consistency. More often than not, only people who were wealthy enough to be able to afford to pay for all the stages in this lengthy process could have the medicine prepared at all. Since these medicines contained no preservatives, they did not last more than a week, which meant that if the patient had to take them over a period of time, they had to be made at regular intervals.

If only, thought Sankunni, he could find the means to make some of the simpler medicines, even on a very small scale ... He considered opening a chit fund, a popular way in those days of making money. But he knew he would be considered too young to run it and that people would refuse to put their trust in him. He asked his father whether he would lend his name to the chit fund, simply as an encouragement for people to invest in it, but his father dismissed the idea, certain that the venture would end in disaster.

Unwilling to accept defeat, Sankunni decided to run the chit fund himself. The initial sum he collected was much less than he had aimed at, but this did not deter him. He thought he would use whatever money he made in this way on his favoured project and begin to process medicines. Opposition came from an unexpected quarter: his mother counselled him not to make the mistake of spending money that actually belonged to others on a venture that seemed to her extremely precarious. Further, she warned him that he would be answerable to all the people who had contributed to the fund if it crashed. She therefore insisted that he hand over the whole sum he had collected to her for safekeeping. So strict were her own priniciples where money was concerned that, when the chit fund matured, she returned this sum to her son with the interest due on it.

It seemed to the young man that he was being continually beset by obstacles, but he did not reject his mother's advice. Instead, without telling her, he emulated her example and began to lend small sums of money against the security of jewels that people brought him, as she herself had been doing for many years. His instinct proved right: whatever he earned in this way, together with what little he made from his Ayurvedic practice, added up to a modest capital.

Meanwhile, he also persuaded the villagers to give him very small sums of money, less than a rupee each, and when all this added up to a hundred rupees, he began to make and sell a few medicines, his highest earnings from this venture never exceeding sixty rupees a month. Eventually, both his parents noticed that his perseverance was not without results and contributed some money themselves to his project.

But Sankunni knew he would soon have to stop all these activities, terminate his studies and go away to get his eyes treated since none of the remedies he had tried for his ailment so far had worked. Dr V. Verghese, who was the chief of the government hospital in Manjeri, a town that was not too far from Kottakkal, had an excellent reputation for curing eye ailments. After much deliberation, Sankunni decided to go to him.

In July 1892, he started for Manjeri. The only way to get there was to walk the entire distance of sixteen miles. The day he set out proved to be unforgettable for an unexpected reason. A stranger who introduced himself as Govinda Varier joined him on the way. He seemed very friendly, professed to know many people in Manjeri and offered to help Sankunni once he reached there. As they walked along, talking of this and that, Govinda Varier caught sight of an elegant ring Sankunni had on his finger, admired it very much and asked to see it.

Sankunni took it off at once to show him and the man returned it after looking at it closely.

Trudging along all day, by dusk they came to a little house near a temple. It turned out to be a variam. The occupants were obviously very poor, for it was a dilapidated place, with a leaky roof and filthy floors and walls. There seemed to be no men in the house. Govinda Varier whispered something to the women and signed to Sankunni to come in. He went in unsuspectingly. It was very dark inside; no lamps had been lighted because, they were told, there was no oil to pour in them. They drank some kanji by the feeble glow of a lamp one of the women brought from the temple, curled up on mats and went to sleep. Exhausted by the long day's walk, Sankunni fell asleep at once.

He woke up in the middle of the night, drenched. The floor and his mat were wet as well. It was raining and water was dripping through the leaky roof.

The women appeared and led them to a room which they said had a stronger roof. Sankunni dried himself hurriedly and found to his horror that his ring was missing. It was pitch dark in the house, so there was no way they could look for it. The women counselled him to wait till morning. Sankunni felt too uneasy to go back to sleep. He got up up at dawn and began to search for his ring. The women suggested very casually that rats might have taken it. Sankunni was very irritated. The quicker he left this place, the better, he thought to himself and left the place hurriedly.

The persistent Govinda Varier caught up with him very soon, however, friendly as ever. Those women are a bad lot, he said to Sankunni, and thieves as well. We should never have trusted them. Sankunni's hopes were kindled again. Why not report the incident to the police then, he suggested. Govinda Varier agreed it was the wisest thing to do and even pointed to a house nearby where, he said, a police constable lived. He offered to go in and talk to him first and Sankunni waited outside patiently. After a few minutes, the older man came out and told Sankunni softly that things did not look good. What if the women said that Sankunni had made improper suggestions to them, that he was trying to foist a case of theft on them because they had not complied with his wishes?

Sankunni realized belatedly that Govinda Varier had played a clever ruse on him and that he had walked into the trap naïvely. Anyway, the ring was lost and he would never recover it. He decided the most dignified thing to do now was to keep quiet, rid himself of the other man's unpleasant company and get to Manjeri as quickly as possible. He learned a valuable lesson from this experience: never to trust people whom he encountered casually.

Dr Verghese examined the young boy's eyes as soon as he arrived and made a diagnosis of a condition then called granular ophthalmia and known in modern medicine as trichiasis, introspection of the eyelashes. The right eyelid had begun to droop slightly and surgery had to be done on it twice before medication could be started. The medication was effective and Sankunni's condition improved in two months: he not only felt better, he could even read comfortably.

Meanwhile, in these two months, the doctor and the young boy had got to know each other well and the older man had grown to like the boy very much. He was therefore reluctant to take the fee that had been fixed for the treatment and young Sankunni Varier had to insist on his accepting it.

Varier had used the time he spent in the hospital to observe the routine there and the manner in which Dr Verghese dealt with his patients. He soon realized that the doctor was a remarkably gifted man, extremely learned in his field and a caring and generous person. His skills were not confined to treating eye diseases, he had acquired a reputation for being able to cure patients who came to him with all kinds of other ailments. He did surgical procedures regularly and successfully as well.

Varier's desire to know more about western medicine grew even stronger as he saw all that was happening around him in the hospital. But if he were to do a course in this subject, he would first have to pass the matriculation examination and then find the means to pay his fees. If only he could stay here as he had stayed at Kuttanchery Mooss's illam, he thought, and have the opportunity to be taught by this talented man as Vasudevan Mooss had taught him. But this seemed an impudent suggestion and he did not dare speak of it to Dr Verghese. He could only long for it ceaselessly inside himself and the greater his longing grew, the more reluctant he felt to leave Manjeri and go back home.

The opportunity he craved with no thought that it would ever be granted fell into his hands like a gift from the gods. The doctor said to the boy as he was about to take leave of him: 'If you want to make vaidyam your livelihood, Varier, you would do well to stay with me here for some time.' The boy was so overcome by emotion that he could scarcely articulate an answer, too near tears to trust himself to speak.

What followed was perhaps one of the happiest stages in young Varier's life, when he became the sole and full-time student of this extraordinarily generous teacher. He found lodgings nearby and soon evolved a routine. He would get up very early in the morning, have his bath, study for an hour or two and drink the kanji made of broken rice that was the morning meal in most Kerala households of the time. At seven-thirty, he would present himself at Dr Verghese's house and they would go together to the hospital at eight.

In the hospital, the doctor would ask Varier to examine the patients who had come that day and give him their medical history in detail. Having been used to this procedure when he was a disciple at Vasudevan Mooss's illam, the boy would go

ahead with the examination and make a diagnosis on the basis
of the knowledge he had acquired through a study of Ayurveda.
If there was something he had missed or had not paid enough
attention to, if he made a mistake of any kind, the doctor
would explain this to him, sometimes re-examining the patient
to demonstrate his findings.

The doctor would then write a prescription and entrust
Varier with the responsibility of handing over the medicines
he had listed in it. Whether the patient was admitted in the
hospital or was to return after a few days as an out-patient,
Varier had to monitor the reactions the medicines had on his
ailment and report them to Dr Verghese. If the patient showed
no improvement with the prescribed medication, the doctor
would ponder over alternatives and discuss them in detail with
Varier.

Varier would leave after the morning session, have lunch
in a small hotel and go to the doctor's house by two. From
two to four in the afternoon, the doctor taught him at home,
using the latest textbooks that had been published. He taught
him Anatomy, Physiology, Medicine and the Materia Medica
in this way. They went back to the hospital at four and stayed
there until six, following the same routine as they had done in
the morning.

A period of study mingled with recreation followed, from
six to nine in the evening. Teacher and student spent these
hours in the doctor's house. He would go over the details of
all the cases they had seen during the day and sometimes take
out a textbook to illustrate a specific point, initiating an
animated discussion. On many occasions, his friends would
drop in on them. The doctor had a lively sense of humour and
would often narrate amusing anecdotes or mimic the patients'
mannerisms or the awkward way in which they had described
their symptoms, making them all laugh.

In addition to all this, Dr Verghese allowed the young boy

to be present in the theatre when he performed surgery and observe him. Slowly, he began to permit Varier to give the patients chloroform and later, to perform minor surgical procedures. Varier would be with him on the occasions when he did a postmortem and the doctor would explain every detail of whichever part of the body he was dissecting to the boy. The doctor also took him along when he visited a patient in his own house.

After Varier had his dinner, he usually read late into the night, conscientiously assimilating the vast and varied aspects of knowledge he had acquired in the course of each eventful day.

Teacher and student observed this unchanging routine through three years. In between, Dr Verghese was transferred from Manjeri to Vadagara in north Malabar, but their schedule was not affected by this change. In the course of the three years, Varier amassed much greater knowledge of the subject than he could have hoped to gather if he had enrolled for a medical degree in a college—knowledge, moreover, that was in-depth and of an extremely practical nature.

At some time during this period, Varier started a sambandham, a contractual marriage arrangement, with a young girl who belonged to the Eranjamanna variam in Manjeri. According to the matrilineal system, this gave him the rights of a visiting husband in her variam. However, this relationship did not find favour with the Varier society in the area and he was obliged to give up the arrangement quickly.

In 1895, Dr Verghese was suddenly transferred to Cudappah, in the Andhra district, and this pleasant stage in Varier's life had to be abruptly terminated. Cudappah was far away from Kerala and Varier was reluctant to leave his parents for such a distant place, for both were growing old. Moreover, as the seniormost male member of the Panniyinpally family, it was he who bore the responsibility for looking after many affairs at Kottakkal. Until now, he had managed to visit Kottakkal now and then and fulfil his duties without too much difficulty, but he would not be able to do this from Cudappah. But more important than all this, he was aware that his destiny lay ultimately in Kottakkal, that everything he had learnt until then would only serve as a means to achieve his primary aim, which he had never lost sight of: the propagation of Ayurveda.

In spite of knowing this with certainty, he was heartbroken at the thought of parting from the doctor, whom he had grown to love like an older brother. He could not restrain his tears all through the night before they were to go their separate ways. They set out from Vadagara in the same train. When Varier got down at the Tirur station, he could not bring himself to speak, his heart was too full and his grief too overwhelming.

5

The Long Period of Waiting

Varier came back to Kottakkal in 1895 with a mind teeming with ideas, determined to improve and modernize the practice of Ayurveda. Because the methods used to process Ayurvedic medicines were so complicated and so dependent on a hierarchy of helpers—those who could identify and collect the necessary raw materials, those who had acquired an expertise in processing them and were familiar with right proportions and correct consistencies, to name a few—Ayurvedic physicians could do little more than actually prescribe a medicine. The lack of experience, the carelessness and ignorance that those who made up the medicines could display, had begun to affect the practice of Ayurveda seriously.

Varier himself once had a salutary experience in this connection when he gave a patient a prescription. The patient had the medicine made up and took it for a month, then came back to tell Varier that he did not feel any better. Varier asked him to take the same medicine for another month, but this time he asked the patient to show it to him after it had been made up. He discovered that his suspicions had been well-founded: certain ingredients mentioned in the prescription had been left out while preparing the medicine, the patient had been none the wiser and the remedy had naturally failed to have the desired effect. Varier realized with increasing regret and frustration that such malpractices would ultimately result in making people lose faith in this ancient system and that the only solution was to find a way to process Ayurvedic medicines under organized and expert supervision.

Having observed and experienced over the last few years how much simpler it was for patients to begin a course of treatment in western medicine, since they could buy medicines ready-made as soon as they were given a prescription, Varier grew increasingly impatient to start processing his own medicines for patients to buy and use, although the idea of selling ready-made Ayurvedic medicines was completely unheard-of at the time. Before his trip to Manjeri he had already tried to do this on a small scale and not been entirely unsuccessful. He hoped he could now extend those efforts and establish an oushadhasala, a recognized centre where he could process and sell Ayurvedic medicines. He knew he would of course have to first find the capital for such a venture.

Meanwhile, he began to prescribe western medicines in his practice, the way he had learnt during his tenure with Dr Verghese. This earned him the displeasure of a person who wielded considerable power in Kottakkal, the thampuran who was then the head of the kovilakam. A petty rivalry lay behind the thampuran's disapproving attitude: the kovilakam physician at the time was a Brahmin who had trained for a while under Kuttanchery Vasudevan Mooss and then acquired a smattering of western medicine. He had been doing quite well until young Varier returned and began to make a name for himself as a reliable physician. Angry that his practice had diminished, he had sought the help of the head of the kovilakam. This apart, Sankunni Varier's father, Rama Varier, was the manager of the same head thampuran's uncle's household. There had been some ill feeling between uncle and nephew in which the straightforward Rama Varier was unfortunately involved. All this meant that the thampuran was not well disposed to Rama Varier and his family and was therefore happy to find occasion to find fault with young Sankunni.

To make things worse, the thampuran reprimanded the young man publicly on the day of Vishu, the Malayalam New Year, when it was the custom for the people of the village to gather at the kovilakam to be given new coins, a symbol of prosperity for the year to come. Not only did the thampuran caution young Varier against prescribing drugs, which he was apparently not properly qualified to recommend, but he also added a threat: 'Be careful or you will find chains on your feet!' Varier refused to be provoked and replied gently that he had only put the knowledge he had gained to the best use he knew. All the same, he realized that in the face of such antagonism, he would have to bide his time to carry out the innovations he so deeply desired to make. And anyway, he still had to find the funds for his project.

For the moment, he took the precaution of explaining to every patient the details of the prescriptions he wrote, making sure they understood why he was using a specific drug and what results it would produce. He also began to insist on being paid in advance for whatever he prescribed. Initially, this led to a sharp fall in the number of patients who sought his advice, for the villagers were not used to such procedures. But as it gradually became apparent to them that his methods of treatment consistently met with success, more and more people flocked to the 'Varier boy' who was proving to be such a gifted physician.

This period proved satisfying for Varier in many other ways, for he was able to find the time to pursue his varied interests. He learnt the aesthetics of poetry, based on the text

of the *Kuvalayanandam Chandrika*, from Killimangalam Krishna
Varier who was staying at the kovilakam. Varier's mother had
already taught him the fundamentals of music when he was a
child. A musician named Perumangottu Krishna Varier used to
come to the variam to teach the women the padams or songs
used in Kathakali. Varier had always loved Kathakali and he
asked Krishna Varier to teach him all the songs in half a dozen
attakathas, the Kathakali performance texts. Krishnanattam, a
specialized dance form which depicted stories of Krishna, was
then being performed regularly at the kovilakam. Varier went
to see Sundaram Bhagavathar, the musician who sang for the
troupe and learnt from him the songs for a number of items
in Krishnanattam as well. Once he had mastered all these
songs, Varier began to sing them along with the musicians who
sang at performances.

He also started to make time to teach during this period.
One of his first students was his young cousin, Kutty Varasyar's
son, Krishnan, who was later to become a well-known poet.
He taught him Vagbhata's *Ashtangahridayam*. He then gathered
a group of students whom he first taught Sanskrit and then the
Ashtangahridayam. Teaching was a passion he never gave up
and he dedicated himself to it throughout his life.

These were days packed with activity. He had his patients,
his music lessons, his own students to teach. The obsessive
desire to find a way to process Ayurvedic medicines was never
far from his mind. And apart from all these, he had his share
of domestic worries.

In 1895, the year he returned to Kottakkal, his Cheriyamma
Kutty Varasyar's second daughter, Madhavi, died. The
astrologers had warned Kutty Varasyar that the Mangulangara
variam was inauspicious, that she would lose one of her
children if she stayed there. So she had moved to a small rented
house in Mangulangara. In spite of this, her daughter Madhavi
had suddenly fallen ill. Sankunni Varier was summoned and he

walked from Kottakkal to Mangulangara the same day to see his cousin. His mother followed. But Madhavi was beyond help by the time they arrived. Her death shattered Kutty Varasyar completely. She and her family had to be taken to Kottakkal.

With the arrival of Kutty Varasyar and her children, the southern variam, the old house that Raghava Varier had built when the Panniyinpally Variers first came to Kottakkal, became too congested and uncomfortable to accommodate everyone. In addition, with its earthen walls and flimsy wooden partitions, it was very unsafe. Young Varier was thinking of rebuilding it when a frightening incident took place that made him hasten this decision.

Varier's mother's little business was flourishing. The jewels that were in her safekeeping and the money she earned from her venture were all kept in a small room in the western wing on the first floor of the house. There was only a partition made of thin wooden planks between this room and the bedroom facing north that Varier slept in. One night, Varier woke up hearing a crackling sound from behind the partition. Thinking it was a cat, he shooed it away and went back to sleep. But the sound started up again. After this happened three or four times, Varier decided to take a look and was just in time to see a thief trying to get at the valuables his mother had put away. Fortunately, the man fled when he saw Varier and the family was spared a disastrous loss. Varier knew he could not delay the rebuilding of this old place any longer.

Once Kutty Varasyar moved to Kottakkal, Varier's father, Rama Varier, found it impossible to manage on his own and went to live with a sister and her children. He would have liked to move to Kottakkal, but the thampuran in charge of the kovilakam was still displeased with him and he thought it unwise to return under such circumstances.

The family decided to demolish the variam that had been

built at Mangulangara, since no one lived there anymore and to use whatever material they could salvage from it for the reconstruction of the variam at Kottakkal.

In 1898, Varier took his mother and his Cheriyamma, Kutty Varasyar, to Rameshwaram so that they could have a bath in the sacred waters and rid themselves of all the evil influences that had brought about Madhavi's death. In 1899, he began work on the new variam and it was completed in 1900. A modest, two-storeyed, tiled house built in the traditional Kerala style around a nalukettu, an open sunken courtyard flanked by wooden pillars, it still stands today, not greatly changed by the passage of time. Once the work of building started, Varier had very little time for his usual pursuits. He found it difficult even to see his patients. But he somehow made time, no matter how hard it was, to teach his students regularly.

Around this time, Varier yielded to family pressure and agreed to marry a girl from the Attoor variam in Deshamangalam. She was not educated but was a soft-spoken, gentle and self-effacing companion.

In 1899, the thampuran who had been antagonistic to Rama Varier died. Rama Varier came to meet the new head of the kovilakam, who was well disposed to him. He was offered the post of manager at the kovilakam and came back to stay in Kottakkal. He built a small outhouse next to the newly constructed southern variam and stayed there. There was already a structure with earthen walls at the spot, which he demolished. He built a small stone house with iron bars on the windows, but did not tile the roof.

Unfortunately, Rama Varier could not stay long in Kottakkal. Age and the onset of physical weakness made it difficult for him to continue his duties at the kovilakam. He returned to Mangulangara in 1901, to his own family variam. His sudden departure and the misfortunes that followed were later attributed to the inauspicious omens that shadowed the house for within a short time of his going away, he sustained a fall and became very ill. Varier, his mother and Lakshmi Varasyar rushed to Mangulangara. Rama Varier survived only a week after they arrived. He died in February 1901.

Rama Varier bequeathed everything he had to his only son, Sankunni. This was contrary to the usual practice—according to the matrilineal system of inheritance, his property should have passed to his sisters and their children. Although it was one of Rama Varier's nephews who had signed as a witness on his will, his other nephews, displeased with their uncle's decision, deliberately stayed away from the funeral ceremonies. Varier did not want to provoke their antagonism. He sold whatever landed property his father had possessed to the thampuran. They agreed that the thampuran would give Sankunni Varier seven hundred rupees and Rama Varier's five sisters and their families two hundred rupees each. Apart from this property, Varier inherited a sum of two thousand rupees from his father and a gold thread that he considered extremely precious, his father's last gift to him.

Rama Varier's funeral rites had scarcely been completed when his son had to face another calamity. Word came that his loved and revered guru Kuttanchery Vasudevan Mooss was gravely ill and not likely to survive very long. Varier was devastated. He had visited his teacher many times after he had come back to Kottakkal, to take his blessing and to meet Aryan Mooss's mother, who had given him so much affection. He could not believe that a great calamity was at hand, that he might not even be able to see his guru again.

Unfortunately, young Varier could not leave as soon as he heard this disturbing news since he was still occupied with the funeral rituals at home. He made ready to leave as soon as he could, walking the whole distance of seventy-two miles, since there was no transport of any kind on that route. All the way to the Kuttanchery illam, he prayed he would find his teacher alive. How could he start an oushadasala to process medicines without his guru's blessing? Would he arrive in time to receive it? Would he be able to see his teacher? Anxiety quickened his footsteps, he knew he was racing against time. Stopping only to snatch some food on the way now and then, he covered the distance in two days.

It was four in the evening when he arrived at Kuttanchery Mooss's illam. God was with him, his guru was still alive. Since he had been travelling and was polluted, he could not enter the house at once. He hurried to the tank, immersed himself in it and rushed into the house, his clothes dripping wet. He first prostrated at Vasudevan Mooss's feet, then stood up and looked at his face. Perhaps his sudden entry had created a stir in the waiting stillness of the room, for his teacher opened his eyes and looked at him steadily for the space of a long minute. A spark moved in the tired eyes, and Varier realized with unbounded happiness that his guru had recognized him. He received the silent blessing those eyes granted him with deep gratitude.

Vasudevan Mooss died at five that evening. Varier often wondered in the years that followed: what if his teacher had died at four and he had arrived at five . . .

But God had not been that cruel. He had his teacher's blessing, his father's fortune, the modest sums of money he had made himself from his practice—the way was clear at last and he could think in practical terms of how and where to build the little medical centre he had dreamed of so passionately, a place where he could examine his patients and they could collect their prescriptions and their medicines at the same time.

6

The Arya Vaidya Sala

Varier bought a small plot of land in Kottakkal for a hundred and twenty five rupees, east of the road that led from the kovilakam to the bazaar. When the thampuran who was the head of the kovilakam discovered that Varier wanted to construct a building on it he raised objections. It took Varier some time to solve this problem. The thampuran's nephew, who liked Varier, had to intervene and get the old man to relent.

The small tiled building that was the germ of the Arya Vaidya Sala that we know today still stands at the entrance to the vast complex that now houses the offices and factory. At the time when it was built, a hundred years ago, its objective and character were unique.

The building was inaugurated on Vijayadashami day, in October 1902. The announcement that Varier had printed and distributed for the function describes it better than any account that can be given of it. The signature at the end of this remarkable document marks the first time he signed his name (Panniyinpally Sankunni Varier) as P.S. Varier, which was how he came to be known for the rest of his life. This is the announcement in full:

ARYA VAIDYA SALA, KOTTAKKAL
AN ANNOUNCEMENT

I do not think I have to explain to anyone the greatness of the Arya vaidyam that we have thought of with such pride from time immemorial as India's particular wealth. Still, Vagbhata has said:

Yaathi halahalatvam cha
Sadyo durbhajanasthitham

That is to say, it is certain that anything kept in a dirty vessel can suddenly turn poisonous. We have to admit that indigenous medicine has begun to suffer serious damage and ill repute since most of its practitioners have, in the recent past, failed to act or make others act in an appropriate manner because of their disrespect for their profession as well as their incompetence and helplessness.

To be so lazy that instead of increasing, even marginally, this wealth that our forefathers have amassed after the hard work of many years—a wealth that is extremely useful and essential for all of us in so many ways that we cannot ignore it, no matter what age we are—we allow it to be squandered away from day to day; to endure without any apparent emotion the ridicule thrown at this system by those who are envious of it or who misunderstand it by attributing to it numerous drawbacks which in fact do not exist: I do not think there is anything more shameful than this.

Although I will now refrain from saying more about the sorry state of most of our vaidyans today lest it become a reason for many to feel displeased, I cannot throw away this opportunity to say at least a few words about the present state of our indigenous drugs.

We have reached a stage where it is generally only those who work for daily wages who now gather, stock, sell, buy, process and use these raw materials, mainly herbs. Not only do they not mix it in the right proportions and at the right time, it has even become a habit with them to make mistakes and confuse even those drugs that are easily available and identifiable. Apart from this, because of a growing lack of familiarity with them, innumerable medicinal plants and roots have now become impossible to identify.

Since outsiders to the system are thus being given total responsibility and vaidyans themselves refuse to take any, not only do people think that the phalashruthi (that part of the formulation that describes the various indications for using a particular drug and its efficacy if so used) is only a series of wordy embellishments, vaidyans themselves are in the process of losing all acquaintance with the medicines they prescribe. For instance, in the formulation of the medicine called 'drakshadi', the ingredient, 'parooshakam' (a Sanskrit word meaning a species of date palm) is usually specified in the prescription by its Malayalam equivalent, 'chitteenthal.' However, if the patient were to query its identity and availability, it would be an enviable situation for a physician to know the true answer and not say, 'Ask those who pluck the medicines!' How can a warrior who knows nothing about the weapon he wields win a war? If all vaidyans become like this, it will not be at all surprising for people to be dissatisfied with them, to lose faith in them.

I have said all this only because I feel that all vaidyans must be familiar with the various kinds of herbs they prescribe; you must not think that I insist that all vaidyans should prepare many kinds of medicines and keep them ready for use. Not that this is not a good thing to do; it is just that it is not possible to do it. Although food, clothes, household articles and so on are things that everyone needs, we all know it would be contrary to the way of the world to try and manufacture each of these things ourselves, besides being impossible.

Therefore, at this moment, it is my opinion that it is imperative that we do not suffer in isolation but that we unite, trust each other, distribute the work we have to do among ourselves and be of help to each other. Vaidyans should organize themselves in a group and form a company that will examine all raw materials thoroughly and see that they are processed with the utmost zeal and attention, making no deviations whatsoever in what the ancient Ayurvedic scientists have prescribed in their texts or in the experience that has been garnered to date. It is my belief that if other vaidyans begin to buy medicines processed in this way, use them properly and conduct treatment in a befitting manner, both groups will enjoy a profit that will equal their effort, that patients will be benefited and people will have faith and satisfaction in native medicine.

This is the special advantage that practitioners of English (western) medicine enjoy. There are numerous shops in all cities to provide them with the medicines and materials they need for treatment. Why cannot we create the same facilities for ourselves? There is no need for me to use the examples of our forefathers here and bore you. Talent does not have to be handed down from parent to child, it can be acquired or learned. While I say with deep sorrow that the time to innovate indigenous medicine according to the needs of the day has already overtaken us, I also take courage in the thought that if we unite and make the joint effort I spoke of earlier, we will still be successful.

The primary reason for the establishment of this Arya Vaidya Sala is the conviction that our greatest duty is to make an effort to seek prestige in the future rather than waste time regretting the past.

Apart from making ourselves ready to treat patients with the utmost attention and care, we have also made preparations to gather raw herbs in the right manner, process them according to the classical prescriptions and sell them at reasonable prices for the convenient use of other physicians and patients.

None of our herbs will be used without being meticulously examined, and none of our products will be processed without special supervision.

We can state with confidence that there will be absolutely no adulteration in our medicines.

Most of the classical formulations which are in common use will always be available.

Several kashayams (aqueous extractions) will be prepared according to modern methods in order to avoid decomposition.

Most of the ingredients are ordered from distant places to ensure their quality and have been accepted as the best in the world.

Some formulations used in Kerala are made up and sold in other parts of India on rare occasions, but except for the fact that they are much more expensive, they are not any better in quality.

Any formulation mentioned in a prescription given by a vaidyan will be instantly prepared. But such

prescriptions have to be written clearly and their cost
deposited in advance.

We will not leave even the most trivial requirement
unattended. Replies will be dispatched tomorrow to
the letters that arrive in today's mail.

A single trial is sure to satisfy everyone.

Kottakkal
16-10-1902   P.S. VARIER

'P.S. Varier was indeed not the first to undertake largescale
manufacture and sale of indigenous medicines,'[5] says the
historian, K.N. Panikkar. N.N. Sen and Company had started
producing medicines on a large scale in 1884, Chandra Kishore
Sen's firm, C.K. Sen and Company in 1898 and Shakti
Aushadalaya of Dacca in 1901. But Varier was certainly the
first to start processing Ayurvedic medicines in Kerala, and the
kashayams (aqueous extractions) to which he refers in his
announcement were being bottled for the first time anywhere.

The Arya Vaidya Sala invited suspicion and adverse criticism
because of its very novelty. The local people could not follow
P.S. Varier's arguments and many of them, including his own
relatives, were pessimistic about the outcome of this strange
venture.

However, it soon became apparent that buying ready-made
medicines had many advantages and the number of people who
went to the Arya Vaidya Sala grew steadily. Varier attended to
every letter that arrived, drafted a reply and dispatched the
required medicine for the ailment in question. Medicines were
dispatched by post as well as by rail. If they had to go by rail,

[5]Panikkar, K.N.: 'Indigenous Medicine and Cultural Hegemony',
*Culture, Ideology, Hegemony: Intellectuals and Social Consciouness in
Colonial India*, Tulika, 1995, p.170.

they were transported to the nearest railway station, Tirur, in a bullock cart and then by railway parcel.

In addition, Varier made every effort he could to keep in touch with all the different kinds of vaidyam currently practised. He visited all the vaidyans in Kottakkal and its neighbourhood, whatever caste or background they belonged to, anxious to keep in touch with varied trends and practices. He considered nothing trivial or negligible, every system had something he could learn from.

The texture of the medicines prepared in the Arya Vaidya Sala had to be absolutely right when they were taken off the fire and had to be carefully tested by an expert: this was something Varier insisted upon. The consistencies of medicines varied according to the prescription. Varier chose his helpers with care. Cheriyamveettil Kunjunni Nair was the first person appointed to work in the Arya Vaidya Sala. He did not stay very long. The next person who came, Pulloor Parangotan Nair, who is really considered the first to have joined service in the Arya Vaidya Sala, stayed with the establishment for many years.

The first person to join the clerical department was T.K. Krishna Menon, known to everyone as Shinnan Menon. He later became the head clerk and then the cashier, worked for many years as a loyal and trusted employee and was appointed one of the trustees in P.S. Varier's will. M. Achuthan Nair, who was to distinguish himself later in a very different role, was appointed as Shinnan Menon's assistant.

A man named Rama Varier, an old friend of P.S. Varier, looked after the supply of the drugs. He made sure there were enough drugs of both varieties—those that could be bought in a shop as well as the herbs that had to be plucked fresh—at all times. There were two foremen who worked with the actual processing, one to weigh the ingredients, the other to check the consistencies as the medicines boiled over a fire fed with coconut fibre. They remained in the service of the Arya Vaidya Sala for many years. P.S. Varier himself supervised every stage of the processing, anxious to make sure that nothing went wrong.

About six months after the Vaidya Sala was started, there was an outbreak of cholera in the region. People had always thought of the disease as a punishment inflicted by the wrath of the Goddess and victims were seldom treated. They were left to die in hundreds. It was the first time since he had learnt vaidyam and started to practise that Varier was brought face to face with a calamity of this nature and he quickly and unhesitatingly seized the chance to prove himself. He flung himself wholeheartedly into a fight against the disease, visiting the sick, ministering to them, consoling them. After a period of testing, he discovered a tablet, the 'vishoochikari' (vishoochika is the Sanskrit for cholera) that relieved vomiting and diarrhoea, symptoms of the dreaded disease. Side by side with whatever treatment he could administer, he counselled the patients, explaining to them that cholera was not a divine malediction, that they could fight it and prevent its recurrence by paying adequate attention to hygiene and health. It was unheard of for a vaidyan of that time to approach patients and talk to them in this manner and the villagers, who were astonished and disbelieving at first, began to accept his humane and generous overtures with gratitude.

His greatest ally through this period was his mother, Kunjukutty Varasyar. Her own mother had been a victim of the terrible disease, so perhaps she understood the risks it presented much better than ordinary people would. Refusing to surrender to the fear that her son might become infected, she encouraged him to go on with his efforts to minister to the ill and dying while she prayed to Venkitta Thevar with redoubled fervour.

Varier wrote and published a booklet on the treatment of

cholera, a subject in which he had gained very valuable first-hand experience. Meanwhile, he continued to be tirelessly active in the Arya Vaidya Sala, constantly looking for new methods to process medicines. Once he had established the Vaidya Sala, Varier realized that ready-made medicines of the kind he made and sold did not indicate the exact dosage for each. Vagbhata advises the physician to work this out on the basis of various factors: the physical and mental condition of the patient, the environment he lives in, the effect that seasonal changes have on his body and so on. P.S. Varier felt that unless a standard dosage was fixed for each medicine, buyers of ready-made medicines would have no idea of how to administer them. He therefore began to prepare a long list that detailed the dosage and method of use for Ayurvedic drugs and also indicated for what disease each would be effective. This catalogue of medicines, the *Oushada Pattika*, was printed and published in 1903. The booklet did a great deal to promote Ayurvedic medicines, since it was simple and lucid and even people who had not had much education could easily understand it.

These were years of intense activity for Varier, and through them a pattern was beginning to take shape. Here was a young man who had grown up in a small village in the interior of Kerala against a background of traditional mores that he had neither actively rebelled against nor rejected. Rather, he had been exemplary in his unwavering obedience to their demands. And yet, no sooner did he start making his own decisions about life than he began to aim at the unusual, dare the unconventional. It was a pattern which was to grow more and more pronounced as the years passed and become one of the most remarkable traits of his extraordinary personality.

7

The Dhanvanthari *Magazine*

The years immediately following the establishment of the Arya Vaidya Sala in 1902 were filled with stimulating activity. The Vaidya Sala was not simply the realization of a personal ideal for P.S. Varier nor was it a mere commercial venture. It was part of his passionate desire to make Ayurveda a dependable and efficient system of health care, easily accessible to everyone. The establishment of the Arya Vaidya Sala at Kottakkal fulfilled only an infinitesimal fraction of this dream. He wanted similar vaidya salas to be established everywhere in Kerala. He wanted all the vaidyans to meet regularly and exchange ideas, formulate plans for the future. He wanted Ayurveda to emerge as the best and most reliable health care system available to people in the country.

An opportunity for action came his way quite soon. An Ayurvedic physician named Vellanasserry Vasudevan Mooss decided to open a vaidya sala called the Arogya Chintamani in Kuttoor. The inauguration was a festive affair and all the well-known vaidyans of the day were invited to it. P.S. Varier was requested to preside over the function since he had been the first among them to open a vaidya sala. Varier reiterated the ideals he had spoken of in his announcement when he had opened his own vaidya sala—that vaidyans should unite and work for the propagation of Ayurveda, modifying and modernizing its concepts and practices to suit the needs of the times. Many who were present agreed with him. An association called the Arya Vaidya Samajam was formed in response to the need they all felt for concerted effort. They decided before they parted company that day to meet at least once a year and Varier invited them to hold the first meeting in Kottakkal.

This function, held in January 1903, lasted two days and was conducted in a shamiana put up next to the Arya Vaidya Sala building. Many vaidyans attended this meeting. Varier was appointed the secretary of a newly formed committee. One of the first decisions the Arya Vaidya Samajam took at this meeting was to hold an examination in vaidyam every year for students who wished to study the subject. Those who passed the examination would be given certificates.

These years were not devoid of domestic problems for Varier. He had been staying in the outhouse of the southern variam, the small building that his father had stayed in briefly when he came back to Kottakkal. According to the astrologers, the bad omens it had been said to have still clung to it and the family was advised to rebuild it and lay a tiled roof. By 1905, Varier was able to do this with the money he had made from the sale of medicines.

The pawned jewels that his mother kept in her safe custody, the money she made from these transactions and all the money that belonged to his mother and his Cheriyamma, Kutty Varasyar, used to be kept in the old outhouse. Once it was demolished, these things were moved to the main house for safekeeping and were directly in Kunjukutty Varasyar's care. She continued to keep them in her charge even when the new and stronger building was ready, for, deep down within herself, she was still not sure that her son was not spending more than he earned from the sale of his medicines! Sensing her unease, Varier asked no questions. He hoped that she would realize, in her own time, that he was not the unsound businessman she took him for.

This practical and sensible woman did have the opportunity to witness her son's success and rejoice in it, but she did not have the good fortune to live long enough to experience its rewards. She had a severe attack of dysentery towards the middle of 1906, became very ill and did not respond to treatment. She died within a month of falling ill. She was only sixty-eight.

P.S. Varier was in indifferent health himself at the time, but this did not deter him from performing all the rites connected with his mother's death with diligent affection. Kunjukutty Varasyar had been a steady, curbing influence on him all her life and had always restrained him when he became too impetuous. He had never rebelled against the control she had exercised gently and firmly over him and had learnt a great deal from her, especially how to manage money. It was because of her that he had realized that the family assets had to be kept separate from whatever he earned by his own efforts, a principle that he adhered to rigidly all his life. She had never been demonstrative or indulgent, but he had taken strength from her quiet affection. He knew her passing away would leave a great void in his life.

In 1907, he conducted the ceremonies for the first anniversary of his mother's death on an even more elaborate scale than he had conducted her funeral rites, spending close to two thousand rupees, the turnover in the Vaidya Sala that year having been excellent.

In the course of the death anniversary celebrations, he gave two of his earliest teachers the gurudakshina, the gift every student lays at a teacher's feet when he asks for his blessing

before going forth into the world. P.S. Varier had not given
Konath Achutha Varier, who had taught him the first chapters
of vaidyam and Killimangalam Krishna Varier, who had taught
him Sanskrit, their gurudakshina. He gave them both handsome
gifts on this occasion and requested them to bless him. Varier
discovered then that an old man named Mannil Kunjikrishnan
Nair, who had looked after him when he was a small child,
had come to attend the function. Varier laid gifts and a handful
of sovereigns at his feet and prostrated before him, asking for
his blessing as well. The old man, who had not expected
anything like this, was completely overcome and gave him his
blessing, tears streaming down his face.

Not long after this function, Varier had to endure the grief
of another death. His wife had been pregnant on the occasion
of his mother's death anniversary. In October 1907 she had a
stillborn child, following which she fell gravely ill. She died in
a few days.

With this calamity, Varier felt that he had no more close
ties. His parents had gone, and now his wife. He had no
children. All his personal bonds had been severed. The only
people he could think of now as family were his Cheriyamma
Kutty Varasyar and her children.

With his mother's death, he had become the real head of
the Panniyinpally family as well. He had been its head in name
since he was twelve, but his mother had looked after all its
affairs with such efficiency that he had been spared any anxiety
on this account.

At the time of his mother's death, the family property
amounted to a few pieces of land and the money earned from
the pawned jewels, a business that had consistently flourished.
This money added up to Rs 2594, 8 annas 3 pies. Apart from
this, there was money that his mother, his Cheriyamma and he
himself had put into this business and the jewels that had
belonged to his mother.

Varier knew that his Cheriyamma had to now take his mother's place. He therefore handed over the money and jewels to her and asked her to look after the affairs of the family and the household with the help of her son, P.V. Krishna Varier. He said he would help them if they needed extra funds at any time. In 1908, he took Kunji Varasyar and her daughter, Lakshmi Varasyar, to Rameshwaram for a dip in the sacred Sethu river to cleanse themselves of whatever evil influences the planets had been exercising over their lives. While he was in Rameswaram, he took the opportunity to perform funeral rites for his father as well.

For years, the family had needed some land for two requirements. One was a bathing tank of their own. The village tanks were always crowded and the members of Varier's family had long begun to feel the need for a private tank. They had experienced the lack of one acutely when Kunjukutty Varasyar died and they had had to request a neighbour for the use of their tank to perform the funeral rites. In 1909, Varier managed to buy a small piece of land about fifty feet away from the variam and he spent close to a thousand rupees to build a small, neat tank there for the members of the household.

The next task before him was to find a cremation-ground for the use of the family. Not to have a cremation-ground of their own was considered shameful for a respectable family. Varier bought a small property to be used for this purpose. He then constructed a wall around the variam. For all these requirements, he used the money he had earned for himself from examining patients. There were a few small sums of money owing to his mother from minor transactions she had had outside Kottakkal. He recovered these amounts and bought land with them for the family.

Varier used the taravad money for the family's needs but kept aside the proceeds from the Arya Vaidya Sala to develop its facilities. These were principles he never deviated from and he even came to believe eventually that he had been destined to a solitary state in life so that no other commitments would distract him from adhering to them.

Varier's first effort at compiling a catalogue of Ayurvedic medicines describing their nature, their efficacy with regard to different ailments, their dosage and so on had met with considerable success. He thought he would extend this information and write a more detailed book on the subject. He therefore started to work on a book called the *Chikitsasamgraham* in Malayalam. It was published in 1907 and subsequently went into many reprints. It has been translated into many other Indian languages as well as into English. The book details the uses of different kinds of Ayurvedic drugs, the methods of use and dosage and describes common diseases, various methods of treatment used in Ayurveda and the regimens prescribed while they are being done. Later editions include information on the Arya Vaidya Sala—its location, hours of work, the requirements to be fulfilled when medicines had to be prescribed by correspondence, the fees for consultation and so on.

In 1910, Varier wrote a booklet called the *Oushadha Nirmana Kramam*, which set out the formulations used to process different medicines. Such formulations had been the secret possessions of vaidyans until then. Varier realized that they would be lost to posterity unless they were documented, and set himself the task of doing this.

In 1903, not long after the inaugural meeting of the Arya Vaidya Samajam, it was decided to bring out a magazine called the *Dhanvanthari*, dedicated to vaidyam, from Kottakkal. P.S. Varier was the editor and his cousin P.V. Krishna Varier, Kutty Varasyar's son, who was by then a well-known literary figure, the manager. The magazine survived for twenty-three years and was a treasure house of varied kinds of information on a multitude of subjects. The contributions ranged from scholarly articles on specific diseases and their treatment to amusing warnings on the evils of moustaches!

The *Dhanvanthari* reported regularly on the activities of the Arya Vaidya Samajam. It published the syllabus, the rules and regulations and the question papers set for the examinations run by the Samajam and announced the results.

The magazine dealt with many other subjects besides the Samajam, many of them related to vaidyam, and developed a unique flavour all its own. It had a picture of Dhanvanthari, the god of healing, on the cover, with a Malayalam verse below it, an invocation to the god written by Kerala Varma Valia Koyi Thampuran, one of Kerala's great literary figures. It then set forth its aims, declaring itself 'the only Malayalam magazine that discusses everything needed to maintain the health and prolong the life of a human being,' and invited contributions on any subject related to medicine. The articles were therefore not restricted to Ayurveda: there were essays on homeopathy, siddha and western medicine, some of which were translations. Sometimes they would have a series of articles on one particular topic that ran into multiple issues—like P.K. Varier's articles on the alimentary system and diabetes, P.S. Varier's on 'Surgery in India' (which featured six pages of illustrations of instruments used in ancient Ayurveda), a series on the duties of a mother by Mayyanattu V. Ikkavamma, another series on the Department of Indigenous Medicine in Travancore. The editors often invited opinions or discussions on controversial subjects, provoking lively discussions.

There were occasional contributions in verse. A serial translation of Vagbhata's *Ashtangahridayam* into Malayalam verse by P.M. Govindan Vaidyan ran into many issues. The editor solicited comments from readers on this endeavour and there were prompt replies, many of which praised the lucidity of the translation. Ashtavaidyan Thaykkat Divakaran Mooss, to cite one of the critics, remarked that although the translation had not in any way deviated from the original in meaning, great care had been taken to render it in pure Malayalam and that not even a stray Sanskrit expression had crept into it.

Each time a new vaidya sala was opened in Kerala, Varier reported the news in the *Dhanvanthari* and offered the management his congratulations and good wishes. He encouraged vaidyans to send queries to the magazine, which were promptly answered, and invited articles recording unusual experiences.

Varier himself contributed articles regularly. Besides writing on medical subjects, he wrote articles that described the policies and objectives of the magazine. In 1904, the editorial announced that the magazine would send out a questionnaire to readers: the aim of the *Dhanvanthari*, it said, was to modernize aryavaidyam, to introduce innovations compatible with the changing times they all lived in. The *Dhanvanthari* was anxious to find out whether readers thought this was necessary. They undertook to publish the replies. There were three questions to be answered:

- Is aryavaidyam or indigenous medicine as it is practised now entirely flawless and worthy of acceptance? Yes or no; state your reasons.

- Is it necessary to modernize aryavaidyam? If it is not, why do you think so?

- If you feel it is necessary to modernize aryavaidyam, what do you think are the measures that have to be taken?

The questions distinctly echoed Varier's own preoccupations at the time. Leading intellectuals and vaidyans of the period sent in their replies, which were published in the magazine. Many of them felt that aryavaidyam had declined because it was not being taught or practised properly and that patasalas or educational institutions with good teachers had to be established in order to train good vaidyans. Some recommended that the

royal houses of Travancore, Cochin and Kozhikode be
approached for financial help in this matter. It was generally
felt that aryavaidyam had always been and would always be
worthy of acceptance, but that it had to evolve and be taught
by competent teachers in good institutions. Some of the
responses pointed out that Ayurveda had never made room for
mutual discussion and that it had to do so now in order to
progress. There were readers who felt that students of indigenous
medicine had to be taught western medicine as well as
aryavaidyam, especially Surgery, Anatomy and Physiology;
that scientific methods of processing medicines had to be
demonstrated to them and that the wealthier sections of
society had to contribute towards the achievement of this
important goal. It was obvious from the replies to the
questionnaire that P.S.Varier's ideas had received strong support,
but the funds to plan and build even a single educational
institution of the kind all these intelligent readers proposed
were still not forthcoming.

Meanwhile, the Arya Vaidya Sala continued to maintain
steady progress. The *Dhanvanthari* announced the sales figures
from time to time. From Rs 1033 in 1903, the amount of
money made on the sale of medicines rose to Rs 2600 in 1904,
Rs 4600 in 1905, Rs 5475 in 1906, Rs 15,000 in 1910, Rs 24,000
in 1911, Rs 29,000 in 1912, Rs 32,000 in 1913, Rs 37,400 in
1914, reaching a total of Rs 52,675 in 1918.

A long and very lively debate was carried on in successive
issues of the *Dhanvanthari* on the question of whether the life-
force was situated in the heart, the head or the navel. The
magazine announced in 1913 that they would carry articles by
various participants in the debate highlighting the principles of
aryavaidyam and western medicine side by side. Varier himself
closed this debate in the October 1913 issue of the *Dhanvanthari*,
in an article entitled 'Our Opinion'. Summing up the varied
viewpoints expressed in the articles, he concluded with a

characteristic comment: 'There is no point in our trying to convince others that there are truths in aryavaidyam which do not in fact exist. Nor is there any use in trying to hide the defects it may have. To endeavour to grasp correctly what is true and to gather what we lack from other schools of medicine or from experience, to try and convince the people and the Government that "our vaidyam can hold its own with any kind of medicine practised in the world today": only such an effort will bring us success and this is something we should all know.'

In 1914, Varier wrote a series of articles in the *Dhanvanthari* on 'Western and Eastern Medicine'. These articles argued the cause of Ayurveda passionately and convincingly, emphasizing its intrinsic value and worth. Varier declared that Ayurveda was of divine origin; that the Creator, Brahma himself, had laid down the principles of Ayurveda in a hundred thousand shlokas called the *Brahmasamhita* and that his son, the great king Daksha and the Aswini Devas had learnt it from him, reciting it by rote. Either because they wanted to simplify this text, or because they needed, with the passage of time, to make changes in it, later sages like Atreya rewrote the *Brahmasamhita* in a modified form after discussing the changes with other great rishis. This was how the *Charakam* and the *Sushrutham*, the two great ancient texts that embody the essence of Ayurveda, came into being. But even these modified texts became too difficult for ordinary human beings to master and neither was sufficient by itself. This was the time when Vagbhata appeared on the scene. He summarized all the older texts and compiled a new one based on them, the *Ashtangasamgraham*, which he later reworked and made even more concise: the *Ashtangahridayam*, which is what vaidyans in Kerala ultimately adopted as their textbook. Varier explained that Vagbhata had used not only Brahma's text but also one that Shiva had compiled. The main difference between these two was in the nature of the medicines they prescribed. While Brahma favoured medicines extracted from roots, plants and herbs, Shiva recommended those made from metals and minerals.

Varier dates the use of both kinds of medicines in India from the time Vagbhata published his text, in which he judiciously combined both sources. Varier felt that this ancient school of medicine which existed in India in the pre-Aryan period gradually moved westwards, undergoing many changes as it travelled, modifying itself to different climates, new geographical conditions and grew into a western tradition of medicine. If western medicine had grown in popularity in recent times in India, Varier felt it was because the British had brought with them an organized infrastructure to dispense it, because they had superior tools and their ready-made medicines were plentifully available in shops. Moreover, western medicine was an arm of the government, funded and managed by the British Empire.

In spite of all this, Varier pointed out that Ayurvedic physicians were still sought after, particularly in the rural areas. Indigenous medicines did not provoke the severe side effects that many western drugs did. The most ordinary kitchen ingredients like cooking oils, jaggery, cumin seed, milk or sugar—all these could be used to treat common ailments by someone who knew and understood their medicinal value. Varier argued that Ayurveda proposed a routine and diet that were compatible with the Indian climate; that their courses of treatment were devised to suit the seasonal changes in the country; that, above all, aryavaidyam looked at the human being as a whole entity, in whom all the natural factors had to be evenly balanced. He concluded the series by reminding his readers that India was as rich as it had always been both in its wealth of medicinal plants and herbs and in its collections of palm-leaf manuscripts that contained invaluable texts from ancient times. The study of vaidyam in the twentieth century, Varier insisted, had to be two-pronged: on the one hand, old texts had to be re-read and taught properly to students; on the other, vaidyans had to make themselves aware of what was happening in other schools of medicine, they had to reach out and master what was new in them, to make up for whatever Ayurveda lacked. This was the only way to put aryavaidyam on par with any medical system in the world. The articles are clearly and logically argued; they are at once a brilliant defence of Ayurveda and an appeal to discard what is obsolete in it and inspire it with new life.

The magazine had a few advertisements from time to time, for books or medicines. There is an extremely personalized one published in 1904 for Ksheerabala thailam—this is an oil which is processed over and over again by the same method, a hundred and one times. The advertisement is signed by the Arya Vaidya Sala Manager, P.S. Varier and says: 'Will be ready this month. Many people have placed orders for this thailam, so very little will be left over for sale. This is not easy to make. How much time it takes! What hard work it entails! And what great expense! Available in one-ounce bottles at Rs 5 a bottle and sixteen-ounce bottles at Rs 72 a bottle, it will be sold according to the priority of application for purchase.' There were advertisements for spectacles with four glasses, imported directly from Bilathi (England) to protect the eyes from the glare of sunlight; for a booklet on the best ways to increase beauty and health and live longer.

The *Dhanvanthari* had lighter aspects as well. It gave curious bits of information under the heading, 'Editor's Notes'. An American was declared to have isolated a 'lazy germ' which made students lazy and was attempting to find a remedy for it! Someone had discovered that moustaches trapped germs and that they aggravated the risk of disease. But rumour later declared that shaving the upper lip was bad for the eyes. Let moustache growers wait until something is certain, cautioned the editor! A doctor had reported that tight necklines and collars caused headaches and grey hair! There were occasional warnings like: people with mouth disease and tuberculosis should not kiss; too much driving would result in the loss of hair and eventual baldness; flying into a temper would increase bile formation! One of the issues announced that the Viceroy had sanctioned a medical college for women in Delhi and Rs 15 lakhs had been granted for it. In the issue dated 10 March 1910, an employee of the magazine raised the question: should women be educated? The answer was yes, and they should be taught vaidyam as well. One of the issues for 1908 reported that a Japanese named Kalajama had discovered a bean called the soya that yielded a special milk which was excellent for use in hot countries. The same issue announced that seven women had passed the Assistant Surgeon grade examination in Madras Medical College.

A trader in Ayurvedic medicines lamented in an article that he would have liked to sell medicines of good quality but that he could not procure them, or, if he did manage to, could not identify them! If he asked a vaidyan, the writer continued, all he would do was quote incomprehensible verses in Sanskrit. The trader appealed to the *Dhanvanthari* to clear his doubts, giving a list of medicines: he wanted to be told where they could be found, what category they belonged to (those found in a shop, or those that had to be plucked fresh) and so on. The magazine published the answers to his queries in a later issue.

There were occasional book reviews. The poet Vallathol's *Arogyachintamani*, with a preface by P.S. Varier and a commentary by one of Vallathol's disciples was reviewed in 1904. The book was written in the form of a conversation between Shiva and Parvathy and the reviewer pointed out that some of the verses were sheer poetry all right, but not very useful to vaidyam! But he hastened to add that this was only one fault among many good points.

Book 4, no.3 of 1908 carried an article Varier addressed to the readers of the magazine on his state of mind about the Arya Vaidya Sala. He confessed that he had been as uncertain of its future as anyone. He had started preparations for the establishment many years earlier and had given himself a testing period of two years. Although he felt that the institution had grown over the years, he thought people in general were still not used to buying medicines or paying for them, that they had no idea whatsoever of the costs of manufacture. They did not understand that medicines processed under the strict supervision of a trained vaidyan could be of a much higher quality than home-made ones and were reluctant to pay the price marked on them. In spite of this, he recorded that sales had gone up considerably over the five years the Vaidya Sala had been in existence. He was anxious to process more medicines and to perfect existing ones. In this article, he also spoke of his intention to establish a patasala to teach aryavaidyam, and a hospital for the convenience of the patients in and around Kottakkal. Since he wanted these to be model institutions, he felt it would take him time to organize them.

The issue of 10 December 1910 set out the rules for this educational institution:

1. There will be four classes and the following subjects will be taught in each class:

    1st class: Yogam (the formulation of compounds of drugs), Chikitsakramam (therapeutic routines, including the administration of medicines) and Gunapatam (the pharmaceutical properties of raw materials.)
    2nd class: *Ashtangahridayam*, first part
    3rd class: *Ashtangahridayam*, second part
    4th class: *Ashtangasamgraham*, *Sushrutham* etc.
    In the last three classes, other lessons will be taught as well.

2. A duration of one year will be needed for each of the above classes.

3. Shastrakriya (Surgery with instruments that penetrate the skin), Yantrakriya (Surgery with instruments that do not go deep into the skin), Oushadha Nirmana Kramam (Pharmacy): as much as is needed of these subjects will be taught during all four classes.

4. All arrangements will be made to teach Shareerabhagam (Anatomy and Physiology) in detail.

5. Only students with a sound knowledge of Sanskrit will be accepted here.

6. If necessary, a separate class will be arranged for those who have no knowledge of Sanskrit.

7. We have no objection to enrolling students of any caste.

8. Fees of eighteen rupees for the First Year, twenty-four rupees for the Second Year, thirty rupees for the Third Year and thirty-six rupees for the Fourth Year will have to be paid.

9. If special classes have to be organized for Sanskrit, a fee of twelve rupees a year will have to be paid for them.

10. A boarding house will be arranged for the convenience of students who require this facility and all the expenses for it will be borne by us.

11. Other rules and amendments will be decided upon as required at the time of commencement.

12. We will not be able to start the institution without at least 50 students or more.

13. We appeal to everyone to help us in whatever way possible with funds.

Arya Vaidya Sala Manager   P.S. VARIER
Kottakkal

The boy Sankunni's intense and obstinate longing to found an institution where students could dedicate themselves completely and whole-heartedly to the study of Ayurveda had not weakened with time—on the contrary, it had grown stronger, more articulate, and was taking a clearer, firmer shape.

On 16 August 1913, P.S. Varier addressed a special article to the readers of the *Dhanvanthari*, which was now eleven years old. It spoke of the pitiful state of aryavaidyam. Practitioners of western medicine had maintained progress because they kept re-examining established tenets and evolving new ones. 'If we close our eyes and tell ourselves that all our ancient principles are true, we will not advance a single step. The *Dhanvanthari* is aimed at propelling us towards progress,' he declared. He said the magazine consistently tried to find meeting points between aryavaidyam and western medicine—if aryavaidyam was better in certain aspects, it was inadequate in the areas of Anatomy, Surgery and Chemistry and steps had to be taken to acquire a more accurate knowledge of these subjects.

Varier wrote an article a few months later drawing the attention of readers to the Medical Registration Bill presented for consideration in 1913, which threatened to put all practitioners of indigenous medicine without a qualification out of practice. If vaidyans were going to be told that their knowledge of Anatomy was defective and inadequate, they had to respond by trying to correct this situation, find ways to learn what they did not know, he said.

This was followed by a spate of articles that reiterated this conviction—notably Varier's own, entitled 'A Mighty Effort', which argued that the establishment of a Patasala where students could equip themselves with sound knowledge and a degree was the only solution to the threat that loomed over aryavaidyam. There were two articles by A.D. Harisharma, a well-known scholar and critic, who pleaded for adequate

measures to be taken before calamity struck and felt that
students who did a course in vaidyam had to be proficient in
both English and Sanskrit in order to understand the texts in
those languages.

On 17 August 1914, P.S.Varier announced the beginning
of the war, which he described as a terrible one. He told
readers of how Germany had backed Austria and attacked
Belgium, of how England had joined the war. An editor's note
announced that everything imported from England for the
manufacture of medicines would go up by thirty per cent. In
October 1914, he addressed his readers again. This time, he
spoke of the Arya Vaidya Sala and the progress it had made.
Not only were the sales good, medicines now went from
Kottakkal to Madras, Madura, Tirunelveli, Chingleput, Trichy,
North Arcot, Coimbatore, Mysore, Hyderabad, Bombay,
Calcutta, Delhi and Benaras in India and to countries like
Burma, Ceylon and Africa. Very often, it was a Malayali who
had gone to these countries who first spread the word about
Kottakkal to his compatriots; later, the people there began to
write and ask for medicines on their own. When the Arya
Vaidya Sala was first opened, Varier said, there had been
complaints that the medicines were too expensive. But their
quality had commended them in course of time. He feared that
costs would now go up with the war—already the prices of
ghee, oil, milk and firewood were rising. Varier concluded by
saying that the Vaidya Sala did not believe in being arrogant
about its success: the blessing of Lord Dhanvanthari and of the
people of Kerala had made it what it was.

In 1916, Varier wrote an article entitled 'The Truth About
Us', in which he summed up the efforts that had been made
for Ayurveda. The Arya Vaidya Sala, he said, had treated poor
patients free and charged rich ones. There had been no
complaints and many vaidya salas had been opened in Kerala
after the one in Kottakkal was established. The *Dhanvanthari*

had tried to serve the cause of Ayurveda by explaining its principles to its readers and by consistently encouraging the writing of articles dealing with all schools of vaidyam—articles, moreover that both lay people and students of vaidyam could follow. The Arya Vaidya Samajam had furnished a platform for serious discussions on how to improve Ayurveda. The Samajam had arrived at a decision to found an educational institution that would train a new generation of vaidyans. The Medical Registration Bill, Varier said, had reinforced this decision, but the project continued to be delayed because the funds they needed had not materialized. Varier felt strongly that they could not delay any longer. A patasala had to start functioning, possibly in Kozhikode.

The *Dhanvanthari* magazine thus served as a mouthpiece not only for the Arya Vaidya Samajam as a whole, but also individually for vaidyans and intellectuals who wished to take part in the current discussion on how best to propagate Ayurveda. The questions Varier repeatedly raised in its columns and the answers they engendered certainly convinced him that he was not alone in realising the threat hanging over Ayurveda and in accepting that the best solution lay in organizing regular courses for vaidyans. If he was disheartened because the protracted discussions dragged on from 1903 to 1917 without any hope of this solution taking shape, Varier did not say so. On the contrary, the *Dhanvanthari* of 16 August 1916 affirmed his decision to spend his own money and start a patasala, for which, he annouced, he had a place ready.

8

The Parama Shiva Vilasam Nataka Company

P.S. Varier had learned the fundamentals of music from his mother. In 1907, he wrote an article in the *Dhanvanthari* which said that it was not enough for vaidyans to learn the contents of textbooks, that they had to be proficient in the arts as well, particularly in music. The article went on to justify this statement. Varier declared that a knowledge of tala, the rhythm-pattern or beat in music, was absolutely necessary in order to examine the pulse, for instance. The normal beat of a pulse followed the rhythm of the eka tala; the slightest change in the sequence of the beats meant that something was wrong. Similarly, he argued that a knowledge of svara, pitch, helped to diagnose irregularities in the heartbeat. Courses of Ayurvedic treatment had to be conducted at a certain pace, which could be defined in terms of tala: if they were performed slower or faster than this pace, damage could result. The correct processing of medicines, once again, depended upon a quick reaction to the difference in the sounds inside a covered vessel as the medicine simmered in it: the knowledge of svara could identify the slightest change in such sounds and gauge the exact point at which the brew would be ready to be taken off the fire. Apart from this, Varier praised the therapeutic effects of music in his article, its power to soothen and gladden the mind.

Before the Arya Vaidya Sala was opened, while Varier still had the leisure to pursue the study of music, he spent time learning to sing the songs that accompanied performances of Kathakali and Krishnanattam.

Audiences of this period appreciated these performances, but most of the professional musicians who sang for them were ignorant of the meaning of the words of the songs. If the songs were in Sanskrit, they paid little attention to the pronunciation and let the words run into one another in such a way that they made no sense to anyone who knew the language. However, when P.S. Varier learnt these songs, he had, with his passion for perfection, trained himself to enunciate each word clearly, attending to the poetic form. But these efforts were completely lost on his listeners, who had grown so used to hearing garbled, indistinct versions of the songs that they actually thought Varier was singing them wrong!

Word reached the Samoothiri, the Prince of Kozhikode, that the young vaidyan who had dared to learn such specialized kinds of music and sing them for performances was distorting the words. Krishnanattam was then a royal prerogative of the Samoothiris and only they could authorize a performance. The Samoothiri had already heard of the culprit, since Sundaram Bhagavathar, the singer of the Krishnanattam group in the east kovilakam at Kottakkal, who had taught P.S. Varier the songs, had sought permission from his employer before he had begun to teach the young man. Anxious to find out whether the rumours were true and curious about Varier's talents, the Samoothiri gave orders for Varier to sing in his presence. Those who had accused Varier of mispronouncing the words waited eagerly for him to be chastised. But they were disappointed. The Samoothiri was a Sanskrit scholar and could follow every nuance of the language. Nodding his head in deep appreciation as Varier sang, he commended him warmly, remarking how much more enjoyable the music sounded when the singer understood the words.

After this incident, Varier had not really exploited this talent since he had meanwhile become preoccupied with many other things: the Arya Vaidya Sala, the Samajam, the *Dhanvanthari* magazine and the many demands they imposed on his time. However, circumstances in his own establishment offered him a chance to become deeply involved in music again and he was quick to take it.

Summertime was a season of comparative idleness in the Arya Vaidya Sala. Raw materials were scarce and not many indigenous medicines could be processed. How could workers who relied on the Vaidya Sala for their livelihood be dismissed simply because they did not have enough work over a certain period? It was against Varier's principles to do so and he cast around for ways to keep his employees usefully occupied in this season. A group of young men in Kottakkal had just then abandoned the effort to form a theatre group under the leadership of P.S. Varier's cousin, P.V. Krishna Varier and disbanded it because they could find only one Malayalam play, T.C. Achutha Menon's *Sangeetha Naishadam*, to produce and were tired of repeating it. Varier was aware that some of his workers had been part of this group, that there were men who could sing and act among them. Why not, he thought, organize a theatre group of his own and get his employees to stage plays, maybe new Malayalam plays? They would then have work in these idle months and, in addition, all Kottakkal could enjoy what they produced.

And so the Parama Shiva Vilasam Nataka Company was born in 1909. It was no coincidence that the initials of the company were his own: P.S.V.

This was a period when Tamil drama was very popular in Kerala—troupes from Tamil Nadu came there regularly to perform Tamil sangeeta-natakams, musical plays in which actors both sang and spoke their parts. The Malayalam stage had hardly any repertoire of its own. P.S. Varier decided to remedy this situation, to write Malayalam plays that Kerala audiences would appreciate and have them performed. The first play he chose was Kalidasa's *Shakunthalam*, which he translated into Malayalam. He set the songs he composed for it to music, chose actors to play the parts and trained them to sing as well as to act. The play was performed successfully and was the only one he wrote whose text was published, first in the *Kavanakaumudi*, the poetry magazine edited by P.V. Krishna Varier, and then as a book in 1913. The book has a preface by K. Ramakrishna Pillai, the fiery editor of the *Svadeshabhimani*, a newspaper which was confiscated by the British government. Varier rendered the play in simple Malayalam that anyone who spoke the language could understand.

In his foreword to the published edition, Varier explains the guidelines he used while translating the play. He wanted the language to echo the spoken idiom of his own region, central Kerala, to avoid heavy or complicated phrases and to preserve the original meaning. He took care to make the songs short and simple, comprehensible to everyone and capable of evoking the emotion of the context they were set in. He wanted the speeches to be short and relevant as well. He had decided to keep some of Kalidasa's verses that were easy to understand in their original poetic form, while he had transformed others into songs. These were broadly the guidelines he was to follow for the numerous translations and adaptations that followed the *Sangeeta Shakunthalam* and for other plays that he wrote.

Ramakrishna Pillai's preface to the published edition of the play[6] particularly mentions the excellence of P.S. Varier's translation:

> ... the book is not just a translation. In certain places the translator has inserted sections which are not in the original. Sections which are in prose in the original have been changed into poems or songs ... I am not sure what justification Varier has to offer for making such changes. I have heard it said that one of his objectives is 'to write a model play which will suit the current trends in Kerala'. This must be his justification, then. If someone were to ask whether he has a particular need or right to do such a thing, I have an answer for that. It is not enough to say that Varier is a sahridayan in the fields of music and literature, one who truly appreciates these arts; he is also someone who has gained immeasurable experience in both. Besides, he has unbounded interest in drama and acting. As a result, thanks to his enthusiasm, a theatre association and a drama company have been functioning in Kottakkal for the last few years, funded entirely by him ...
>
> The translation is not a word-by-word one, it is completely free. The prose, the poetry and the songs in this translation follow the style of the Malayalam language, using Malayalam words that are familiar to Malayalis ... Varier has to be congratulated for having made efforts no one else has made so far in the matter of composing the songs. There are no less than one hundred and seventy songs in all the seven acts together. It is no small matter that the composer has expended

---

[6]Vaidyaratnam P.S. Varier: *Sangeeta Shakunthalam*, Norman Printing Bureau, Kozhikode, 1913.

great effort in giving each song a different style, a different mode. Of the hundred and seventy songs and the sixty-odd verses, a hundred and thirty-seven songs are in the style of Tamil or Malayalam drama and have been composed to fit the context; two or three are in the style of kathakali songs from performaces like the *Nala Charitham*; eleven are in the manner of the Mysore javalis and the remaining nineteen in the manner of kirtanas or compositions in Carnatic music.

P.S. Varier says in his own preface to the second edition of this play that he incorporated certain changes on Ramakrishna Pillai's suggestion, especially in the matter of shortening the play. The *Sangeeta Shakunthalam* became one of the most successful items in his repertoire.

Varier's next efforts were translations from Tamil, the sections of the *Harischandra Charitham* (The Story of Harischandra) set in Kashi and the cremation-ground. Pazhayannoor Narayana Bhagavathar helped him with these translations since P.S. Varier did not know Tamil himself. This was followed by Varier's own translation from the Sanskrit of the section of the *Harischandra Charitham* set in Ayodhya.

The plays were first performed on a stage built adjacent to the hall that served as a store for the medicines in the Arya Vaidya Sala. They generally started at nine at night and went on until about two in the morning, or sometimes later if it was a long play. An artist named A. Narayana Pisharoty was appointed in 1912 to prepare backdrops, settings and stage props that would make the plays more attractive to spectators.

Around this time, a patient named Govinda Pillai came to P.S. Varier from Travancore for treatment. Varier discovered that Pillai loved theatre and was very knowledgeable about it. With his help, Varier taught his troupe two more plays, *Sadaram* and *Madanasena Charitham*. Together with T.C. Achutha Menon's *Naishadham*, he now had plays for thirteen consecutive days—*Shakunthalam* was acted over three days and *Sadaram* and *Naishadham* over two days each. Meanwhile, Narayana Pisharoty had fabricated the props and settings. Varier decided it was time to take the troupe out of Kottakkal to as many places in Kerala as he could.

In 1912, the troupe performed outside Kottakkal for the first time, in Tirur. They collected about ninety rupees that evening. Although the troupe had a succession of young managers from its inception, it was Varier himself who really supervised the performances in these early days, even outside Kottakkal.

M. Achuthan Nair, who had been appointed as assistant to Shinnan Menon in the Arya Vaidya Sala, proved to be an able actor, an expert in the role of a king, a 'raja-part' as it was known at the time. The first music teacher appointed to train the troupe was Shoolapani Varier from Chunangat. Later, Chidambaram Venkitarama Bhagavathar took over from him. Shivarama Pisharoty played the mridangam. Shekhara Panikker, a talented actor himself, was appointed to teach the actors, but P.S. Varier preferred to train them himself whenever possible and managed to make enough time for this task, no matter how busy he was. Eventually, he kept apart two sessions a day for them, between ten and eleven in the morning and between seven and nine in the evening, a timetable that he tried to adhere to no matter how busy he was.

The *Ramayanam* contributed many plays to the troupe's rapidly enlarging repertoire. Using Thunchath Ezhuthachan's Malayalam rendering of the Sanskrit *Adhyatma Ramayanam*, a text that is widely read and deeply loved in Kerala, Varier wrote the *Paduka Pattabhishekham* (The Coronation of Rama's Sandals), the *Sugreeva Sakhyam* (The Contract between Rama and Sugreeva), the *Lanka Dahanam* (The Burning of Lanka) and the *Ravana Vadham* (The Killing of Ravana). He tried to retain Ezhuthachan's original verses wherever he could, setting

them to music, choosing with care the ragas he thought would
suit the mood of each. Initially, these four episodes were done
as different plays on four consecutive days. Later, he condensed
them into a single play, the *Sampoorna Ramayanam* (The
Complete Ramayanam), to be performed in one evening.

In 1913, P.S. Varier went to see a patient named Subbayya
Shetty in Mangalore. While he was there, he saw a Kannada
performance of the *Prahlada Charitham* (The Story of Prahlada).
Fascinated by the play, he wrote a Malayalam version and had
his troupe perform it. By now, the troupe had begun to
perform regularly all over Kerala. Varier made it a rule that the
performances in each place began with the *Prahlada Charitham*
and ended with the *Sampoorna Ramayanam*.

Varier also wrote plays which were adaptations of the
Mahabharatham. The episodes he chose were the *Pandava
Vanavasam* (The Pandavas in the Forest), the *Ajnathavasam*
(The Pandavas in Disguise), the *Draupadi Vastrakshepam* (The
Disrobing of Draupadi) and the *Daksha Yagam* (The Yaga of
Daksha). He also selected the most dramatic episodes in the
long *Nala Charitham*, (The Story of Nala) and condensed them
into a play that could be performed in one evening. He used
Unnayi Varier's well-known Malayalam text for this play,
retaining the original verses wherever he could, as he had done
for Ezhuthachan's *Ramayanam*.

The songs in the earlier plays were heavily influenced by
Carnatic music, since that was what Varier had studied and was
familiar with. Later, noticing the growing popularity of
Hindustani music in Kerala, he sent one of his musicians north
to study their melodies and wrote Malayalam songs set to these
airs. Krishnan Nair, the brother of the actor Achuthan Nair,
was sent to Thanjavur to study dance so that appropriate
dances could be incorporated in the durbar scenes in plays.

When they went outside Kottakkal to perform, the Parama
Shiva Vilasam troupe also fulfilled the role of a publicity agent

for the Arya Vaidya Sala. On Varier's instructions, the artists
made curtains that carried the legend, 'P.S. Varier's Bhageeratha
Prayathnam' and drawings of the medicine bottles sold in the
Vaidya Sala. This drew attention not only to Bhageeratha's
heroic endeavour to bring the Ganga down to earth but also to
Varier's determination to make known the medicines he
manufactured and their excellent quality.

Varier looked after his troupe with great care when they
toured, according them as much attention as he might have
given his children. Accommodation was always arranged for
everyone in the same place and a cook and necessary kitchen
equipment were taken along to provide their meals. He
discouraged the performers going out alone when they were in
strange places, lest they spend their time drinking or visiting
prostitutes and showed no compunction in punishing actors
who had broken rules repeatedly. But Varier was no tyrant,
nor was he ever judgemental. Once a complaint was brought
to him that Achuthan Nair, one of the best actors in the
troupe, drank heavily and associated with women of ill repute.
'Will he play his roles better if his character is good?' retorted
Varier. Whenever his goal was complete perfection, he
overlooked details he considered irrelevant.

K.K. Aroor, who worked in the Parama Shiva Vilasam
Drama troupe from 1919 to 1937 and later acted as the hero of
the first Malayalam talkie, *Balan*, describes the amenities P.S.
Varier granted every member of the troupe:[7]

> For six months, from the month of Edavam (May-
> June) to the month of Thulam (September-October),
> all the members of the drama troupe stayed in
> Kottakkal. They learned new plays, or whatever else

---

[7]Aroor, K.K.: 'Parama Shiva Vilasa Nataka Company', *Souvenir of Vaidyaratnam P.S. Varier's Centenary Celebrations*, 1969, pp.98-9.

each one wished to learn: Carnatic music or instruments like the harmonium, the mridangam, the fiddle, the veena or the flute. Sri Vaidyaratnam took great interest in arranging all kinds of amenities for everyone. Accordingly, he bought many members of the troupe whatever instrument they needed. Apart from this, he arranged driving lessons for many of them and procured them licences when they finished. The great man's aim in doing this was to ensure that everyone would have a livelihood, like driving a vehicle or giving music lessons, in case they wanted to leave the troupe. In addition to this, those who had the inclinition to learn Sanskrit were taught the language and then encouraged to study vaidyam in the Patasala without paying fees.

The members of the troupe enjoyed every kind of convenience in their accommodation in the Vaidya Sala. There were buildings to house them, rooms for everyone, a cot, a chair, a table. The salary itself might have been small, but if the salaries of that time are compared to those of today, it is certain that no one enjoys today the kind of pleasant life and happiness we all had. Besides our salary, we were given two excellent meals a day, coffee morning and evening, ten mundus a year, eight towels, two shirts, a gift on our birthdays, new clothes for Onam, a gift of money for Vishu, an umbrella and shawl every three years, the fare to go home twice a year, living expenses for parents or guardians who visited us, their return fare and new clothes for them as gifts. If we were ill, we received free treatment and whatever oils we needed free of charge . . .

The drama troupe attracted many performers outside Kottakkal who came seeking employment. Meanwhile, in Kottakkal, there was always a constant exchange between the Arya Vaidya Sala and the drama troupe. A full-fledged troupe with props and stage settings required many hands and the employees of the Vaidya Sala took varied duties in their stride, transferring amicably from their jobs in the kitchens or the office by day to helping with the productions in the evenings or acting in them.

In Kozhikode, Varier used the Town Hall for his performances until 1923, in which year he had some difficulty in hiring the premises at the time when he needed it. He decided to build his own hall in Kozhikode and the P.S.V. Hall, which still stands, was inaugurated in 1924 next to the Kozhikode Arya Vaidya Sala with great fanfare and a performance of the *Sangeeta Shakunthalam*. When it was not in use for staging his plays, Varier let it be used free of charge for whatever event the people of Kozhikode pleased.

The troupe toured the entire length of Kerala, from Kannur, Talasserry and Vadagara in the north through Kozhikode, Tirur, Manjeri, Perintalmanna, Pattambi, Ottappalam, Shoranur, Palakkad, Thrissur and Kodungalloor down to Perumbavoor, Moovattupuzha, Vaikkom, Pala, Kottayam, Changanasserry, Thiruvalla, Chertala, Alappuzha and Thiruvananthapuram in the south. Apart from the clamorous applause the performances received everywhere, many of the principal actors were awarded gifts and medals by local dignitaries in the towns where they performed.

An amusing incident has been recorded during the troupe's first visit to Perumbavoor. There was a large group of Tamil Brahmins in the area and they could not believe that a Malayalam-speaking troupe could really perform good plays, since Tamil drama troupes had been holding unchallenged sway for many years in Kerala. They therefore decided to boycott the evening's performance. Incensed, the Nairs in the area took a decision in revenge that they would not give the

Tamil Brahmins any help in the future or participate in any of their activities. This could have had serious consequences, since the Nair community in this area was very influential. The Tamils hastily withdrew their boycott, attended the performance and actually enjoyed it very much!

Mannath Padmanabhan, a social reformer and the founder of the Nair Service Society, was of great help to the drama troupe in the various places they toured.

Varier took particular interest in supervising the arrangements for stage effects, especially in the mythological plays. With the advent of electricity, he was able to achieve amazing and spectacular effects that delighted his audiences. For instance, when Hanuman arrived in Ravana's court, he would twirl his tail discreetly with one hand, pulling it gently out under him and raising it until it formed a seat so high that he could look down regally from it at Ravana on his throne! Krishna would dance on the five-headed serpent, Kaliya, manipulating the strings behind the painted tin sheets that were the serpents' heads so that the bulbs fitted on them flashed on and off. Finally, the tired, defeated serpent would collapse and throw up, emitting a series of sparks from its mouths. Krishna would burst out from a backdrop, twirling his discus, and release a length of cloth that would whirl around Draupadi endlessly. Hanuman would stand poised at the highest point of the stage and leap in an instant across the entire stage propelled by a concealed wire.

Varier somehow found the time to plan and supervise all these painstaking projects in addition to the demands the Vaidya Sala made on him. They added one more dimension to his activities, moving him into yet another area where he could exploit his talents, plan innovative techniques, organize a new series of events.

Thanks to the zeal of a dedicated member of the family, the manuscripts of the plays have been neatly re-copied into notebooks which have been laminated and are available for perusal in the Arya Vaidya Sala Library. There are twenty-nine of them. *Nandanar Charithram* (The Story of Nandanar), *Satyavan Savitri Charithram* (The Story of Satyavan and Savitri), *Sati-Anasuya, Kandi Raja, Manoharan* and *Krishna Leela* are in Tamil. *Pavizhakkodi, Parsi Lalithangi, Sadaram, Lanka Dahanam* (The Burning of Lanka), *Ravana Vadham* (The Killing of Ravana), *Gulebakavali, Draupadi Vastrakshepam* (The Disrobing of Draupadi), *Keechaka Vadham* (The Killing of Keechaka), *Sampoorna Ramayanam* (The Complete Ramayanam), *Nallathangaal Charithram, Sangeeta Shakunthalam, Valliyammal Charithram, Nala Charithram, Pandava Vanavasam* (The Pandavas in the Forest) in two parts, the episodes of *Paduka Pattabhishekham* and *Sugreeva Sakhyam* from the *Ramayanam* as two separate plays, *Kovilan Charithram*, the episodes of *Ajnathavasam* and *Daksha Yagam* from the *Mahabharatham, Harischandran* and *Prahlada Charithram* are in Malayalam.

Of these, *Prahlada Charithram*, all the adaptations based on the *Ramayanam* and the *Mahabharatham* and the Ayodhya section of the *Harischandra Charitham* were plays Varier himself wrote (parts of the last were translated from the Sanskrit). The sections of the *Harischandra Charitham* set in Kashi and in the cremation-ground were translated from the Tamil, so were *Nallathangal Charithram, Manoharan, Allirani Charithram, Gulebakavali, Parsi Lalithangi, Parijathapushpa Haranam* and *Kovilan Charithram*. Apart from these, the company included plays written by others in its repertoire, like *Sangeetha Naishadham, Sadaram, Rukmangada Charitham, Saranjini Parinayam* and *Valliyammal Charitham*.

Varier speaks, in the preface to the second edition of *Sangeeta Shakunthalam*, published in 1936, of how the company was taught Tamil plays from 1928 (this is evidently after the arrival of A.C. Achuthan Nair, a talented actor who came from Tamil Nadu) and of how they stopped learning Malayalam plays for a while:

We now regularly perform a dozen or so Tamil plays, like the *Krishna Leela*. But this is not our final objective. My aim in allowing these Tamil plays to be taught was to gather as much knowledge as possible from Tamil drama in order to modernize Malayalam drama. We now have some good actors for those plays as well. This revised edition of the *Shakunthalam* is being brought out as the first step in the endeavour to further modernize Malayalam drama.[8]

Ragams are indicated in the script for each song. Sometimes only the names of the ragams are mentioned. Often, there is an indication that a song has to be sung in the style and tune of a popular song of the period—this could be a well-known composition in Carnatic music or a popular song that everyone knew. Occasionally, there are Kathakali padams (the songs used in Kathakali performances) sung in the Kathakali style or verses from the *Ramayanam* that P.S. Varier has set to music. A.C. Achuthan Nair speaks of how diligently Varier worked to find the appropriate ragam for the mood and situation that a particular lyric described and how pleased he always was when he achieved what he had wanted.[9]

Sanjayan, Kerala's famous humorist, heaped extravagant praise on Shekhara Panikker, one of the most talented actors in Varier's troupe after he witnessed a performance by him:

The occasion when Sanjayan laughed a truly happy laugh, the kind that brings tears to the eyes, took place last Thursday night. It was provoked by that uncrowned emperor of Kerala actors, the life and soul of the P.S.V. Drama Troupe, Shekhara Panikker . . .

Ten-year-old Sanjayan had once watched without blinking his eyes while Shekhara Panikker, acting as

---

[8]Ibid, p.xxi.
[9]In a personal interview with A.C. Achuthan Nair.

the king of thieves, careful to make sure that not a single bell fastened to his feet made the slightest sound, committed a dozen massive robberies with a skill that made the audience hold its breath . . . It was to see all this again that Sanjayan arrived on Thursday night at nine o'clock for a performance that would start at nine thirty, as greedy as a gourmand going for a feast . . .

That night, Panikker was Moodhashikhamani, the simpleton in *Sadaram*. It was then that Sanjayan realized that the Moodashikhamani's role had to be played by an extremely skilful actor. No make-up on the face, no clothes to conceal the body. And he had to play the role of a sixteen-year-old! Imagine the guts of that sixty-three-year-old man! Have any of you seen the eyes of that fearful form that sprang out of a pillar as Narasimha? I have seen them and shuddered with fear. They are Panikker's eyes. But from where did he bring this expressionless, lacklustre dullness into them when he transformed them into Moodhashikhamani's eyes? How could this empty-headed, idiotic smile diffused over his features have replaced the concentration on Hanuman's as he lunged forward to leap over the ocean? From which firm could he have ordered this voice that sounded like stone grating a glass surface? Who taught this man a flat-footed swan's gait? I will never know. And there is no use asking Panikker: he will just laugh.

Even the Manager of the company calls him 'Master' (can Sanjayan call him that as well?) Many have given Master gifts and medals. Sanjayan's only wealth is the ink in his pen. Of what use is it to splash two drops of that in the ocean over which Master leaped? . . . But Sanjayan says, and it is the truth: those who have

eyes must watch Panikker act. Those who have a soul
will praise him ... Bravo![10]

P.S. Varier must have been happy to read that passage, written
in 1935. It would have marked a moment of real satisfaction,
the knowledge that he had succeeded in his endeavour. For,
although the Parama Shiva Vilasam Nataka Company had
been initially conceived as a group that would engage employees
who had no work in the lean seasons in pleasant activity, it
had very quickly exceeded the modest range of that objective.
It had turned into an expression of Varier's involvement in the
cultural aspects of Kerala's ethos and was to extend into other
domains besides drama, remaining one of his major concerns
throughout his life.

---

[10]M.R. Nair (Sanjayan): 'Shekhara Panikker', *Sanjayan*, Vol. I,
Mathrubhumi Printing and Publishing Company, Kozhikode,
pp.146–47.

9

Widening Horizons

With the continued progress in the processing of medicines, the requirements for opium, ganja and spirit increased. A licence was necessary to stock more than a prescribed quantity of these substances. It was a period when the excise officers in the country had great power and authority. Most of the senior excise officers were British and had little consideration for the manufacture of what they thought of as indigenous and therefore inferior brands of medicine.

From 1902, when it was started, to 1906, the Arya Vaidya Sala did not face any serious difficulty in this connection. In 1906 it became obligatory to have a licence in order to buy or stock these substances. Accordingly, Varier applied for one. Within a few days of his doing so, the Excise Inspector, an Anglo-Indian, appeared at the Vaidya Sala to find out whether he had any unlicensed substances in stock.

There were, in fact, small quantities of opium, ganja and spirit in the Vaidya Sala for which Varier had just applied for a licence. The Inspector was incensed when Varier explained that he had filed an application and not yet received a reply.

'Only practitioners of western medicine are entitled to apply for licences,' he said angrily.

A court order arrived instructing Varier to explain why he had stocked these substances without a licence. Varier went to Kozhikode, where his mentor, Dr Verghese, now worked. The doctor tried to intervene with the District Collector, but was told that in an excise case of this kind, Varier would definitely have to pay a fine. All Varier could do now was prevent future incidents by obtaining a licence as quickly as possible.

On the day of the trial, the excise officers waiting in the court were sure that a person of Varier's stature would have engaged skilled counsel. But Varier arrived there alone, with no counsel to argue his case. Encouraged by this, the Anglo-Indian Inspector piled one accusation upon another, confident that the victim would receive the punishment he deserved.

The court asked P.S. Varier: 'Do you have anything to say?'

'It is true,' said Varier, 'that I had five tolas of opium in my possession. It was ordered from Powell and Company, Bombay. We had ordered ganja as well, but they said they could not send it to us without a licence. Since they had withheld the ganja for want of a licence and sent the opium, I presumed that it was not forbidden to keep opium in my possession.' Varier handed over the documents to prove this statement.

Anyone could store five tolas of opium without a licence in the Bombay Presidency at that time; only three tolas could be stored in the Madras Presidency. Powell and Company had sent Varier five tolas mistakenly, forgetting this difference in the permitted weights. The court found Varier not guilty. The Inspector was infuriated. Varier was charged a nominal fine of five rupees.

Thanks to the certificate that Dr Verghese had given Varier stating that he was qualified to practise western medicine, the District Magistrate took the trouble to make a detailed enquiry into the matter and eventually gave Varier a licence for opium. It took many years and countless applications, reminders and complaints for the licence for spirit to be issued.

By 1909, Varier found that he had to spend more and more time in the Arya Vaidya Sala and that, because of the demands of the *Dhanvanthari* magazine and the drama troupe, he needed space for himself away from the variam. He therefore put up a building ·next to the Vaidya Sala. He had a large bedroom for himself on the first floor and the ground floor was used as a packing area and storage space for medicines.

Both the building which housed the Arya Vaidya Sala and this later one (which is now the administrative office) are still in use and their original structure has been left untouched, though additions and alterations have been made internally. The Vaidya Sala—a modest, tiled building with a rough floor of red country tiles—is now a dispensary. On the left is the little room where Varier used to see his patients. The compounder occupied the central portion, where patients went to get their medicines. Besides dispensing medicines, the compounder also dressed ordinary wounds and administered Argerol drops to all those who came with conjunctivitis in the season when it was rampant in the village—this was part of a tradition that Varier had learnt when he was with Dr Verghese. On the right was a room to store the medicines. At the back of this was a long L-shaped room where there were fireplaces for the processing of medicines and enough space for packing them.

When P.S. Varier's new living quarters were ready, the hall downstairs (which now houses the finance department) was turned into a packing room. Medicines were bottled and labelled here and, if necessary, packed in wooden boxes for dispatch to places outside Kottakkal. There was a post office by then in Kottakkal; Varier records its being opened in the *Dhanvanthari* in 1908. So only railway parcels had to be taken to Tirur. The medicine bottles were sealed with corks and the words, 'Arya Vaidya Sala' and its emblem were embossed on them. Initially, Varier imported bottles made of green-tinted glass from Germany, hexagonal in shape, with full and half ounces marked on them on two sides. Later, he began to buy bottles supplied by local Muslim traders.

A flight of stairs leading from this packing hall terminated in a landing where there was a large window. The landing opened into a big room which Varier used as his bedroom. There was an ordinary spring cot on one side and a punkah was obviously suspended from the other side for its hooks can still be seen. There was a small room just off the hall, where copies of the published edition of the *Sangeeta Sakunthalam* were stored; there was also the kind of simple toilet that was found in all Kerala houses of the time.

At first, Varier used to go home to eat but this proved inconvenient. For some time, food was sent to him from the variam. A cook, Kottur Rama Varier, was employed as time went on, so that Varier did not have to leave the office building at all. It was his home from 1910 to 1929.

As he grew older, the thought that after his time, there would be no one to perform his parents' annual funeral rites began to haunt him. If he could go to Gaya and perform the shraddha rites for both of them there, according to tradition, their souls would require no further rituals. In spite of a whirl of activities that left him little time for travel, he managed to make a trip in 1912 with his Cheriyamma to Gaya. He felt deeply at peace when he completed the rites, his last duty to his parents.

It was during this period when Varier began to stay on his own that a group of people, some of whom were paid employees and some of whom were friends, started to gather around him—a group that was to stay with him for all the years to come, loyally safeguarding his interests.

One of the people who was closely associated with P.S.Varier from the beginning, giving him his whole-hearted support and help in everything he did, was his cousin P.V. Krishna Varier, Kutty Varasyar's only son. Eight years younger than P.S. Varier, Krishna Varier as a child had always looked up to his older cousin. When he finished his studies in Sanskrit, he had been P.S. Varier's first student and had learnt the *Ashtangahridayam* from him. However, Krishna Varier's passion was for literature, particularly poetry, rather than for vaidyam. He took English lessons, did the upper primary examination and then joined the Kerala Vidya Sala, a school in Kozhikode, where he did his matriculation examination. Even as a schoolboy, he showed a keen interest in literary activities and contributed articles and poems to local magazines.

In 1909, Krishna Varier became the editor of the literary journal, *Kavanakaumudi*, which had until then been published from Pandalam and which he moved to Kottakkal. Many poets who later became renowned published their first work in this journal. Krishna Varier himself had by this time become a poet of repute and was known as 'Kavikulaguru', the guru of the poet-race. Apart from the *Dhanvanthari* and the *Kavanakaumudi*, he also published an economics magazine called *Lakshmivilasam* and another one on agriculture called *Janmi*.

However demanding his literary activities were, Krishna Varier was P.S. Varier's loyal and able assistant in all his activities as well. It was when the *Dhanvanthari* was started that Krishna Varier really came into his own: he worked as its manager for twenty-three years, collecting articles, writing his own, translating articles and notes from the English, discussing current trends and events with vaidyans and doctors and transcribing them and, of course, printing and publishing the magazine. He participated enthusiastically in the establishment of the Arya Vaidya Sala and the Arya Vaidya Samajam; it was he who often accompanied the drama troupe on its visits to places outside Kottakkal and who looked after its affairs until the trustworthy Shoolapani Varier became its manager.

K.V. Shoolapani Varier was another sincere and loyal worker on whom P.S. Varier learnt to rely heavily over the years. He joined the Parama Shiva Vilasam Natakam Troupe when he was ten years old. He first learnt to play the mridangam and was later appointed cashier of the troupe. In 1919, he took over as the manager, after a succession of fairly well-educated managers who had seemed to have the necessary qualifications for the post but who proved inept and unreliable. Shoolapani Varier did not even know how to write. Diffident and nervous at being offered such a responsible post, he asked P.S. Varier whether he would be able to hold it for any length of time. But Varier had no such doubts. 'Will you do as I tell you?' he asked Shoolapani, who answered, 'Yes, I will.' 'Then everything will be all right,' said Varier confidently. Varier himself taught Shoolapani his letters and trained him to look after the affairs of the drama troupe. Shoolapani Varier fulfilled his duties with such dedication and proved so dependable and trustworthy that, over the years, he gradually took over the management of almost all of P.S. Varier's interests.

Gentle and infinitely patient by nature, Shoolapani Varier never lost his temper and never spoke ill of anyone, no matter how acutely he was provoked. It is said that his assistants, particularly P.T. Sridharan Nair, an actor with a mischievous temperament, would pull his chair away from under him as he was working in an attempt to make him lose his temper, but he would not protest. He was very vulnerable though, and easily hurt. Varier grew to have so much faith in him that he would not entertain any remarks against him. Someone who did not realize this was foolish enough once to bring a complaint about Shoolapani Varier to P.S. Varier. He listened quietly, then said: 'Never say anything against Shoolapani to me again. I'll have you beaten black and blue if you do!'

A.C. Achuthan Nair[11] was another of this group of people who was very close to P.S. Varier and the story of the bond that he forged with Varier is quite extraordinay. In 1921, at the age of eleven, he joined the Madura Balameenaranjini Sabha, a Tamil drama troupe for young boys, directed by Jagannatha Iyer, and distinguished himself as an actor playing women's parts. The well-known actors, M.R. Radha and Nawab Rajamanickam were part of this troupe. Touring through centres in the Tamil Nadu like Madras, Thanjavur and Nagapattinam, young Achuthan won numerous medals and prizes.

Achuthan came to Kottakkal in 1926 seeking treatment from P.S. Varier. There were no microphones in those days and continual singing and speaking aloud had weakened his lungs. He had developed a painful cough and breathlessness and the harmonium player in his troupe, a Keralite named P.S. Menon, had advised him to go to Kottakkal. He was so ill when he arrived that he could not sing even one song completely.

He underwent treatment for three months but was not very much better. Varier suggested he stay for three more months and he improved considerably during this period. Varier asked whether he would like to stay in Kottakkal and join his troupe and the boy accepted.

When they heard that he had worked with a Tamil troupe, the actors of the Parama Shiva Vilasam troupe wanted the sixteen-year-old boy to teach them a few Tamil plays. Achuthan was worried. He had none of the scripts of the plays that he had acted in with him. But he did have an excellent memory and had followed every production with such attentiveness that he knew all the parts. Writing out the Tamil dialogues in the Malayalam script, young Achuthan managed to teach the troupe the *Krishna Leela, Nandanar Charithram, Satyavan-Savitri, Sati-Anasuya* and *Meerabai.*

Achuthan soon realized what a proficient director P.S. Varier was, what a gift he had for choosing the apt ragam for each song in a play, how sensitive he was to shifting moods and to the potential of a situation and was proud to be part of such a talented troupe.

But in three years' time Achuthan became restless and dissatisfied with acting. He began to read philosophy and grew increasingly fascinated with the idea of giving up worldly pleasures and becoming a sanyasi. He attended bhajan singing sessions in the Ramakrishna Ashramam in Kozhikode and was persuaded by Padmanabha Menon, a friend he made there, to renounce his career and go away to the Himalayas. He chose what he thought was the best day to leave, the day after the celebrations for P.S. Varier's sixtieth birthday in 1929.

But Achuthan had underestimated Varier, who discovered his absence at once. Varier made enquiries, was told the young man had gone to Tirur and sent his manager, Shoolapani Varier, to bring him back.

'Why did you go away?' Varier asked the unrepentant Achuthan.

'Because I don't like theatre. It's useful neither for this world nor the next.'

'Bring me your horoscope,' was Varier's answer. Varier could read horoscopes and had great faith in them. He studied Achuthan's for a while, then told him he was destined to be a vaidyan. The boy was speechless with amazement: how could he consider becoming a vaidyan when he did not even know Sanskrit? Varier did not think this was a serious obstacle, he declared he would begin teaching Achuthan the language at once.

Achuthan spent the next three years learning Sanskrit. Once he had taught him the alphabet and the basic texts, Varier moved on to the study of the Bhagavad Gita as an example of kavyam—for the other world, he explained! It is your karma to learn the Gita, a punishment for having run away! He took up the great poems, the *Magham* and the *Naishadham* only after they had completed the Gita.

Once he had completed the study of Sanskrit, Achuthan attended the Ayurvedic College in Kottakkal, obtained his certificate and became a vaidyan. He continued to act in plays all this while and gave up acting only when the drama troupe was disbanded—at which time he transferred to vaidyam as a full-time profession. He retired as the physician in charge of the Erode branch and now lives in Kottakkal.

Kottur Rama Varier came to work as a cook when P.S. Varier began to stay in the room in the Arya Vaidya Sala. This faithful and dependable employee remained with Varier for many years. There is a story of how one day, in the monsoon season, Varier wondered when he got up in the morning and looked out of the window how Rama Varier would come for work that day, since the street in front of the Vaidya Sala was flooded. He was very surprised when Rama Varier brought him his morning coffee as usual, exactly as the clock struck six. Varier was a stickler for punctuality and no one knew this better than his cook, who had actually swum across the swirling waters to arrive in his kitchen on time! Varier was so pleased that he bought him a wrist watch to show his appreciation. He gifted him another watch for quite a different reason: for being late! Raman Nair brought Varier's morning coffee five minutes late one morning, at five past six. When Varier asked why he was late, Raman Nair said the clock downstairs was five minutes slow and he had gone by the time it showed. Varier's answer was to buy him a new watch with instructions to adjust the time on it to the clock upstairs!

It was during this period that Varier began to write regularly in his diaries. There are eighteen diaries, starting from 1 January 1927 and ending on 29 January 1944, the day before his death. All eighteen are Hoe and Coe's hardbound Premier diaries, with a flap that seals with a press fastener. The entries follow a similar pattern. They start with an account of the routine he maintained for the year that had just gone by. The entry for each day begins unvaryingly with recordings of the outside temperature, Varier's pulse rate and the specific gravity of his urine. They are almost all full-page entries and sometimes spill over to the top of the page, into the small spaces above the date and on its sides. So crowded that the words are often illegible (perhaps because he wrote in a hurry), the entries range over a variety of subjects—from the details of his personal health to world affairs. News of one of the girls in the family coming of age or of another having a baby jostles with bits of information about the drama troupe, what play they did that day and how it was received or whether they had made enough money. He reports on his patients, his visitors, his employees.

On the first of every Malayalam month, he records having a bath in the tank, worshipping in the temples in Kottakkal and examining the omens for the day, to make sure they boded nothing inauspicious. On this day, there is a small drawing fitted into the diary entry—his own horoscope. Varier had studied astrology, could cast and read horoscopes, perform the prasnam ritual to decipher the past and future and work out rites of propitiation or atonement.

There are Sanskrit or Malayalam shlokams on certain pages that he composed himself. There are accounts for earnings and expenditure that are sometimes in code. Often, if it was a day when a feast was served, he would write what he had eaten and remark appreciatively on the vegetable preparation or sweet that had pleased him most.

From these closely-written pages covered in his neat script emerges the portrait of a man who was as meticulous with himself as he was with others, a man who was obsessed with a desire for perfection in not one but many and utterly different things and who, against all odds, strove for and achieved that perfection.

10

The Arya Vaidya Samajam

The Arya Vaidya Samajam continued to hold meetings every year after the first meeting in Kottakkal. From the very beginning, the meetings were characterized by a festive ambience: the venue was always decorated with palm leaf streamers and flowers, and music was played in the intervals between sessions. At the end of each meeting, poets recited mangalashlokams, poems which described the auspicious nature of the function and invoked the blessings of the gods. Often, rose water was sprinkled on the participants as they were leaving and they were each given a lime, a custom marking the close of an auspicious ceremony in Kerala like a wedding or a formal reception.

The decision the Samajam had made during the first meeting to conduct an examination for vaidyans took effect from 1904. Ashtavaidyans and other vaidyans who had until now imparted instruction according to the rules of the gurukula system offered their help and advice on how to conduct the examination. Indeed, the first examiners to be appointed by the Samajam were the head of the Kuttanchery illam, who had succeeded P.S. Varier's guru and Varier himself. However, in the period from 1904 to 1920, only seven candidates passed the junior examination, the Madhyama, and nineteen the senior one, the Uthama. The questions were not easy and perhaps the students were inordinately nervous since they had never been trained or called upon before to take a test like this.

The second meeting of the Arya Vaidya Samajam was held in Kozhikode in 1904. The members made two important decisions: to have the association registered and to open an Arya Vaidya Patasala, an educational institution to teach aryavaidyam, in Kozhikode, for which purpose a committee was formed.

The Cochin government undertook to host the third meeting in Thrissur in 1905, but backed out later. Varier took over and conducted it at his own expense. At this meeting, it was suggested that a way be found for students who had not mastered Sanskrit to learn Ayurveda in Malayalam. A group of ten scholars was appointed to draft textbooks in Malayalam.

The next meeting was held in 1906 in Vadagara, in an old building, the munsif court. Nothing had been done about the proposal to write textbooks in Malayalam. Only P.V. Krishna Varier wrote a series of articles for the *Dhanvanthari* which were later combined and published as a book, the *Aryavaidya Charithram* (A History of Aryavaidyam). Edited by P.S. Varier, this concise book also has illustrations depicting the processing of medicines and a list of instruments which were used in surgery.

The Arya Vaidya Samajam was registered as an association in 1907, when the fifth meeting was held in Pattambi. The *Dhanvanthari* describes this as one of the best-conducted meetings. The venue was elaborately decorated and rose water was sprinkled lavishly over the guests. The members decided at this meeting to hold an exhibition of medicines the coming year.

The sixth meeting was held at Palakkad in 1908. The Elayadath Thaykatt Ittiri Mooss Award was instituted for the student who obtained the highest marks in the Samajam examination. It is significant that this award was instituted by an ashtavaidyan who belonged to the gurukula system for it proved that these vaidyans themselves were aware of the need for radical changes in the methods of study and anxious to support them.

In 1909, for the first time, a scholar from outside Kerala, C. Gopalacharlu from the Ayurveda Ashramam, Madras, was invited to attend the meeting in Kollengode. A committee was appointed to gather funds and organize the details for the establishment of an Ayurvedic College and Dispensary. Gopalacharlu said he would donate a gold medal every year to the student who stood first in the examination held by the Samajam.

The meeting held in 1910 at the Brennan College, Talasserry, hosted a medical exhibition and the halls for the meeting and the exhibition were very grandly decorated. Numerous vaidyans, laywers, journalists, reporters and schoolteachers flocked to the exhibition. Garlands and bouquets were presented to the most important invitees. Eight people brought medicines to be exhibited and the jury examined all the exhibits and gave critical comments on them. P.S. Varier was awarded the first prize for his exhibit. A.K. Kanaran Vaidyan had brought an excellent collection of rare medicinal plants which earned him a special prize. Manakkadan Karayi submitted two old handwritten manuscripts, sections of which were commended as very good. A bigger committee was formed at the meeting, to look into the matter of establishing an Ayurvedic college, since the committee first selected had not achieved anything so far.

In 1911, Varier hosted the ninth meeting in Kottakkal on a grand scale, with an exhibition and festivities. The Deputy

Collector of Malappuram, the 'Tukdi Sahib' as he was known locally, was the guest of honour. He arrived in Kottakkal on the day before the meeting. Next morning, he was escorted to the decorated shamiana in the Arya Vaidya Sala in procession, accompanied by musicians playing the nadaswaram. In his reception speech, he commended P.S. Varier, remarking that he had transformed a location that had been wild jungle ten years ago into an active centre that housed the Arya Vaidya Sala and its offices. He alluded in his speech to an interesting historical coincidence: Rohini Tirunal Eralppadu Thampuran, who had been the second in succession to the royal headship of the Samoothiri family in Kozhikode and had died in 1879 had wanted to establish a vaidya sala in Kottakkal in his lifetime. He had arranged for an indigenous physician to be specially trained in surgery and modern western techniques and actually begun to construct a building when he passed away. The present Arya Vaidya Sala could be seen as the fulfilment of his dream. He went on to say that the examination conducted by the Samajam was not satisfactory. There was no way to screen the candidates who appeared for it or to test their eligibility.

A music recital followed this speech. Medals and prizes were then awarded for the medical exhibition, at which there were exhibits from Madras and Kathiawar as well as from different parts of Kerala. Rao Bahadur Krishnan won a gold medal for his demonstration of surgical instruments and a display of tumours he had excised, with a description of each. Another music recital followed after which the Collector was taken back in procession. On the second day, Varier submitted a suggestion: if the Arya Vaidya Samajam was prepared to spend fifty rupees a month, he could run a patasala in Kottakkal with the money.

The tenth meeting was organized in Mankata in 1912 at the school hall. Not only the hall, but the entire path from the Mankata palace to the hall, was richly decorated and the invitees were led to the venue in procession, accompanied by musicians playing nadaswaram. A sonophone machine, a novelty of the period, played songs and a live music recital followed. A.C. Krishna Varma Raja of the Mankada kovilakam gave the inaugural address. He declared that these annual meetings had been an awakening for Kerala and helped the public appreciate the value of aryavaidyam. He apologised for not having organized a medical exhibition—he had decided against it because Mankada was difficult to access. He lamented the scarcity of dispensaries and hospitals in the rural areas, where both doctors practising western medicine and indigenous physicians were hard to come by. Varier reiterated his plea for the establishment of a patasala and was seconded by several people. Yet another committee was appointed to expedite its opening. After a vote of thanks, the schoolchildren of the village staged an entertainment programme with music and dancing.

These first ten meetings of the Arya Vaidya Samajam certainly succeeded in bringing vaidyans from all over Kerala together to a common venue. The royal families of Travancore, Cochin and Kozhikode, vaidyans, scholars and citizens of importance from various villages and towns—all of them lent their active support and patronage to the Samajam and attended the meetings. The Arya Vaidya Samajam was probably the first body of its kind to involve the participation of members from Malabar, Cochin and Travancore, the three political divisions in Kerala. K.N. Panikkar, Professor of History at Jawaharlal Nehru University until recently, points out that these meetings were also cultural events, accompanied by exhibitions, processions and music and that they evoked the concept of an Aikya Kerala, a united Kerala, 'much before the Indian National Congress organized its first Kerala conference in 1920.'[12]

---

[12]Panikkar, K.N.: 'Indigenous Medicine and Cultural Hegemony' in *Culture, Ideology, Hegemony*, p.162.

The meetings engendered a certain amount of discussion as well, particularly about the decline in aryavaidyam, the need to revitalize methods of study and practice and the acute necessity for a patasala to train a new generation of vaidyans. Royal patronage was offered to host some of the meetings. Varier noted in the *Dhanvanthari* in 1912 that an annotated commentary on Vagbhata's *Ashtangasamgraham* had not been available for a long time and that the manuscript of a commentary written by a disciple of Vagbhata's, named Indu, had been rumoured to be somewhere in Kerala. A senior Cochin prince had eventually discovered the manuscript and his palace vaidyan, Thrikkovil Uzhuthra Varier had painstakingly copied it out. It had then been published by the Mangalodayam Press in Thrissur, with assistance from Appan Thampuran, also of the Cochin royal family. But apart from individual instances of support and encouragement for the cause of Ayurveda like this, no practical move was made towards the founding of the patasala in spite of all the discussion that took place both in the *Dhanvanthari* and at the meetings of the Samajam. This remained one of P.S. Varier's sharpest disappointments all through this period.

A move was made in Madras in late 1913 to pass the Medical Registration Bill, which would distinguish qualified doctors from quacks. It was true that unqualified practitioners who prescribed western medicines had become a menace to the public. But vaidyans who practised indigenous medicine were threatened by the Bill—what if they were declared unfit to practise because they did not hold a qualification? From the wording of the Bill, it was not certain whether the practitioners of Ayurveda, siddha and unani would be affected. At a meeting of the Arya Vaidya Samajam on 6 November 1913, Varier discussed the implications of the Bill with the members. The Samajam decided to wait until the Bill was passed before attempting to take any kind of action.

After the first ten meetings of the Arya Vaidya Samajam, no one offered to host the eleventh and from then onwards, P.S. Varier conducted the annual functions at Kottakkal and bore the expenses himself. In 1914, there was an effort to organize another association called the Keraliya Ayurveda Samajam to which the Cochin royal family promised a sum of thirty thousand rupees. This Samajam decided to establish a vaidya sala in Cheruthuruthy in the Cochin State, near Shoranur, and the foundation stone was laid for it in 1915.

The *Dhanvanthari* of 14 January 1914 carried an article by P.S. Varier entitled 'A Mighty Effort' which pointed out that the Arya Vaidya Samajam had not yet been able to establish a patasala, despite having repeatedly declared its firm intention to do so. Meanwhile, practitioners of Ayurveda equipped with adequate knowledge were becoming more and more scarce. Varier warned his readers that western medicine was therefore in an enviable position at the moment and would be able to take over the country easily, with the modern tools and state support it commanded. Varier called upon the wealthy people of Kerala to help remedy this sorry situation and contribute generously towards an institution to train physicians in indigenous medicine. Once the money was found, it was going to be difficult to find competent and experienced teachers, even more difficult to find dedicated students. The article concluded with an earnest appeal to everyone in Kerala, exhorting them to take note of the plight aryavaidyam was in and do their best to help.

Immediately following this, a general body meeting of the Arya Vaidya Samajam took place at Kozhikode on 25 January 1914 to discuss the organization of an Ayurvedic college and a charitable hospital attached to it. One of the Cochin princes who attended the meeting seemed to have been deeply moved by Varier's article and one more committee was appointed to look into the matter. Varier expressed a hope in the

Dhanvanthari that this committee would work with the Samajam and achieve something concrete. Ravi Varma Koyi Thampuran, a great literary figure, took an active part in the discussion of the formation of the patasala. Indigenous medicine was still studied according to old methods, he said, while western medicine had adopted modern ones. Something had to be done, and quickly. He advocated a five-year course in which Anatomy and Physiology would be taught in English and the ancient Ayurvedic texts in Sanskrit. Only candidates with a basic knowledge of both English and Sanskrit would be eligible to apply for the course. Senior practitioners of indigenous medicine had to be allowed to attend whatever classes they wanted, on payment of a minimal fee, or even without a fee, so that they could update their knowledge and skills. A hospital with a hundred beds and a centre to process medicines had to be attached to this institution. The money for all this, he felt, would flow in if people with nationalist ideals and pride in the ancient tradition of aryavaidyam took over the management. This glowing speech did not produce any results: the patasala stayed a much-discussed and unrealized project.

An ordinary meeting of the Arya Vaidya Samajam held the next month in Thrissur turned out to be unexpectedly festive. Rama Varma Kochunni Thampuran and Appan Thampuran, both of the royal family of Cochin, organized a grand reception for the delegates. Their managers waited at the station with carriages drawn by twin horses to receive the guests, among whom were Samoothiris from Kozhikode, eminent lawyers and representatives of leading newspapers. They were given a sumptuous tea at the kovilakam. A suggestion was made at the meeting to open a patasala in Shoranur under the Ayurvedic physician, Thriprangot Mooss. Rama Varma Kochunni Thampuran pointed out in his speech that he had read P.S. Varier's article and that he felt Varier, who had first put forward the idea of a patasala and had campaigned enthusiastically for it over the years, enduring many disappointments, should be given the responsibility of running it when it was established. There was a feast for the guests at night at the palace and another one before they left next morning. The reporter who was sent to cover the event could not praise the elaborate arrangements for the function and the extravagant hospitality extended to the guests enough!

At the annual meeting held in 1916 at Kottakkal, Varier spoke of how the Arya Vaidya Samajam had been formed in 1903. The first ten meetings, he said, had been conducted on a very grand scale, but, as far as the patasala was concerned, these meetings had not achieved anything. In 1914, at a meeting held in Kozhikode, the Keraliya Ayurveda Samajam had spoken about preparations for starting a patasala and expressed a desire to work with the Arya Vaidya Samajam on this project. However, Varier said, the Keraliya Ayurveda Samajam had later held its meetings without even letting the Arya Vaidya Samajam know about them. Nor had the matter of the patasala been discussed again. Varier had tried to collect money for the college and many wealthy people, including some rich Namboodiri landlords, had promised in writing to make contributions, but had not kept their word. One of them, Varikkasserry Namboodiri, had turned belligerent and even denied having signed a statement saying he would contribute. The Arya Vaidya Samajam had felt that others might follow his example, and decided to file a case against him.

Varier was tired of fighting for a cause that never seemed to make any progress. He had made endless speeches, written innumerable articles, he had argued and pleaded, tried to enlist the financial support of wealthy individuals, all to no purpose. The threat posed by the Medical Registration Bill had convinced him that it was not wise to delay the decision to establish a patasala to train qualified vaidyans. Varier announced that he had decided to go ahead and establish a patasala on his own and that he had already bought the land for it. The fact that the Keraliya Samajam did not seem to have any intention to establish a patasala in the near future was an added incentive for him to carry out his project without further delay.

All P.S. Varier asked for now was the co-operation of the Arya Vaidya Samajam to draw up the rules and regulations for the institution he was going to establish. In October 1916, he opened a branch of the Arya Vaidya Sala in Kozhikode and began to construct a building next to it for the patasala. He organized two meetings of the Samajam in the Kozhikode Vaidya Sala to discuss matters pertaining to the new patasala. Both were chaired by eminent vaidyans: the first by Vaidyaratnam Thriprangot K. Parameswaran Mooss and the second by Ashtavaidyan Elayadath Theykkat Divakaran Mooss. The prospectus (which appeared in the *Dhanvanthari* within a few days of the meetings), the syllabus and the rules and regulations were finalized during these meetings.

A date was set for the opening. For P.S. Varier, this was the long-awaited fulfillment of a dream that thirty years had not tarnished—an obstinate dream that he now knew he *had* to realize if aryavaidyam was to survive.

11

The Patasala

While the Arya Vaidya Samajam had been debating the matter of establishing an institution to teach Ayurveda, practising Ayurvedic physicians had been dwindling in number. The older Namboodiri Ashtavaidyan teachers were reluctant to impart instruction to those who were not of their caste; sometimes they would not even teach the *Ashtangahridayam* fully to students who belonged to other castes. As for the examinations conducted by the Samajam, very few had written them, fewer had passed.

In January 1914, P.S. Varier wrote an article in the *Dhanvanthari* expressing his deep anxiety about the prolonged delay in organizing a patasala to teach vaidyam:

> ... Knowledgeable vaidyans are growing fewer in number. And if even those who are considered knowledgeable now are compared to the old-time vaidyans, we will have to accept that the present day vaidyans do not deserve to be called vaidyans at all. If we make a close search, one or two might be seen to have learnt something from the worthwhile physicians of old. With the next generation, we cannot even hope

to make any effort in this direction. So there is no
doubt at all that the first thing we should do is
establish a vaidya patasala. If the objective of this
patasala is to be fulfilled, it is an indisputable fact that
there must also be a hospital and a centre to process
medicines attached to it. English medicine had taken us
over completely. It has every imaginable kind of tool
as well as assistance from the King. Not only do we
not have any of these, we have to confess now that we
do not even have basic knowledge. There is no need
then to say what the future will be.

This article went on to suggest that the wealthy people in
Kerala should contribute generously towards the capital needed
for this project.

In four successive issues of the *Dhanvanthari* in 1916,
Varier continued his appeal for this cause.

Our aim is to start the patasala as soon as possible and
to run it properly; since it must catch the British
government's eye, it has to be situated in British
Malabar . . . It is not possible to gather the money for
this in fives and tens from people with modest incomes.
Therefore, it is our opinion that wealthy kings,
landlords, noblemen, officials, merchants and so on
should give us their contributions, making no distinction
of caste or religion. A thousand rupees or five hundred
rupees: these are the two amounts we have decided to
appeal for. It will suffice if this sum is given in
convenient instalments: two, four or even five. We
have decided that the worthy people who help us in
this way with money will be consulted about the
administration of the patasala.

The names of various people who had promised to contribute
to the venture followed. But a large portion of the money

never actually materialized. All Varier collected was a meagre five thousand rupees, which he banked in the name of the Arya Vaidya Samajam. It would serve, he thought, as a modest capital.

At the two meetings the Arya Vaidya Samajam held in the newly-opened vaidya sala in Kozhikode, it was decided that Vagbhata's *Ashtangahridayam* would be the basic textbook for the course in the new patasala and that special care would be taken to teach students methods of Ayurvedic treatment like dhara and pizhichil that were unique to Kerala as well as the fundamentals of western medicine. Varier invited suggestions from all those who were present. There were many responses, including some that said the knowledge of both Sanskrit and English had to be a requisite for admission. In the issue of the *Dhanvanthari* that carried the prospectus of the patasala a few days later, P.S. Varier declared that it was his aim to innovate and improve Ayurveda, to make it available and useful to everyone and to convince the British government of its excellence. He felt it was dangerous to start with a syllabus that combined too many traditions and that it was better to concentrate on strengthening India's own system for the moment.

The Arya Vaidya Patasala was inaugurated on 14 January 1917, the day of the festival of Makara Sankranthi, on the fourteenth anniversary of the Arya Vaidya Samajam. The ruling Samoothiri of Kozhikode was the guest of honour at the function.

The guests who had been invited for the occasion, among whom were thampurans from the Cochin royal family and well-known ashtavaidyans, were accommodated at the Kozhikode residence of the Raja of Nilambur. The Samoothiri arrived at the venue at four in the evening along with other members of his family. Varier read a report that gave the details of the Patasala, its aims and curriculum. The Samoothiri then gave a short speech and opened the institution with a silver key. He was shown over the building, which was called the Vaidya Vilasam. He looked at the pictures and statues inside and at some rare palm-leaf manuscripts, then came back to the main hall in front. Varier garlanded everyone of importance.

Forty-two of the sixty applicants were selected for the first course. The only fee they were required to pay was a sum of five rupees. Varier was appointed both Principal and Secretary and he held these posts until his death. The institution offered a four-year course and the diploma of 'Aryavaidyan' after an examination at the end of it, the prefix 'arya' here meaning excellent.

P.S. Varier began to visit Kozhikode once a week to supervise the running of the Patasala. All those who obtained the diploma were to be given special training at the Arya Vaidya Sala in Kottakkal in the processing of medicines and in methods of Ayurvedic treatment.

Two of the first team of teachers to be appointed, P.P. Kammaran Nambiar and P.K. Ramunni Menon, stayed with the institution for many years. In its second year, a doctor who had studied western medicine, a Licentiate in Medicine and Surgery (L.M.S.) was appointed to teach the students Anatomy and Physiology since Varier had always felt that the Ayurvedic system of teaching did not lay enough emphasis on these subjects. This doctor also taught students the elements of modern western medicine.

The first batch of students, numbering fourteen, received their certificate as Aryavaidyans at the twenty-first annual meeting of the Arya Vaidya Samajam held at the Arya Vaidya Sala in Kozhikode in 1921. The certificate, issued by the Arya Vaidya Samajam, was written in Sanskrit and English. It declared that the students had finished a four-year course at the Patasala in the theory and practice of aryavaidyashastram.

'Kalanusrutha parishkarapoorvakam arya vaidya shasthreshu kriyasu cha nipunam paditha.' (That is, they had been taught the science of aryavaidyam in a scientific manner, updated in keeping with the times).

Varier took a keen interest in the curriculum and taught the students Anatomy and nervous disorders himself from the time the Patasala was established until his death in 1944. Varier was immensely popular among the students because he enlivened their classes with witty remarks and jokes. He had a great gift for seeing the humorous side of things and could hand out a reprimand so light-heartedly that the culprit found it impossible to take offence. Aryavaidyan N.P. Krishna Pisharoty speaks of an incident that took place when he was a student in the Patasala. Kammaran Nambiar, who was one of the first teachers to be appointed and who was also the headmaster, used to go home to his village very often. He had built up a fair practice there which he had not abandoned when he came as a teacher to the Patasala. Moreover, there were problems in the family that he often had to attend to personally. P.S.Varier came to know of these frequent absences since, more than once, he found that Nambiar was not at the Patasala at the time when he went there during class hours. The third time this happened, he handed over a piece of paper to Ramunni Menon, who was also a teacher at the Patasala, asking him to give it to Nambiar. To Nambiar's deep embarrassment, the contents of the paper became common knowledge among the students in a few days—they consisted of a witty little verse in Sanskrit on Nambiar's unfortunate proclivity to repeated absence from class!

P.S. Varier used the interest on the deposit of five thousand rupees in the bank as well as the fees he collected from the students towards expenses for the institution, contributing whatever was needed above this from his own funds—that is, from the Arya Vaidya Sala. In the four years it took to train the first batch of students, the earnings from the Arya Vaidya Sala doubled. Varier was therefore rewarded from the beginning by the confidence that he would be able to take care of the expenses of the Patasala with the money he made from the Vaidya Sala.

The years following the end of the First World War in 1919 were extremely grim, especially for the poorer sections of the people. The prices of essential commodities went up steeply. Men who had served temporarily in the Army were thrown out of employment, and there were many who were thus affected in Malabar. Varier had always wanted to build a hospital in Kottakkal which would dispense free medicines and treatment irrespective of caste and creed to people in and around the village. He knew he would now be able to channel a portion of the profits he earned from the Vaidya Sala into this venture. There was no hospital in the village and those who needed free treatment had to walk to Tirur or Malappuram to the government hospitals there. This was perhaps not a really opportune moment to start construction, for, like everyone else, Varier too had been hit by the post-war losses. On the other hand, he knew a large-scale construction of the kind he planned would give regular work to a number of people who were unemployed and starving. Among the many workers whom he gave employment to in this way was a large section of local Muslims who had been in the army during the war and were now unemployed. Their gratitude to P.S. Varier was later to be of significant help to him.

Since there was unrest in Malabar soon after Varier began the construction and he was obliged to suspend the work for almost six months, the hospital was finished only in 1924. It was built on a large piece of land which he acquired on the Tirur-Malappuram road. Once this hospital, which was called the Ayurveda Chikitsasala, began to function, Varier decided to shift the Patasala from Kozhikode to Kottakkal, to a spot next to the hospital, so that students could benefit from the practical experience they would obtain there. The first students who arrived were not at all happy with this move. They missed the urban comforts and conveniences of Kozhikode. Kottakkal was, after all, just another little village in the interior of Kerala. Board and lodging were difficult to arrange, there were no public eating places and no distractions of any kind. The number of applicants dropped sharply. Varier met this challenge unflinchingly. He not only waived the admission fee, he gave stipends to all the students who joined the course in 1925, a measure which promptly brought him more students and which he continued until the institution was stable.

The structures of the Charitable Hospital and the Patasala are preserved in their original state and are still in use, although many new buildings have come up around them. The hospital building, which used to be called 'the bungalow' is elegant and beautifully proportioned. There is a high portico in front with tall wide arches. A flight of steps leads up from it to the central room on the ground floor that was the dispensary and there are two rooms on either side. One was used as a store for medicines, the other was the compounding room. Patients who came for a consultation went straight to the dispensary. It had two doors, one at the front and one at the back. Patients who came for Ayurvedic treatment used the front door, those who opted for western medicine used the back door. The simultaneous dispensation of Ayurvedic and western medicine was a tradition that Varier followed as a consequence of the long and intensive internship he had done with Dr Verghese. Varier himself used to dispense mixtures based on prescriptions he had learned during his apprenticeship with the doctor. He gave these mixtures his own names—for example, a mixture given to cure fits was called 'bhoothasamhara dravakam', a mixture that destroys bhoothams, the evil spirits that cause fits. 'Agnideepa dravakam' a carminative mixture, cured indigestion, quelled the 'agni', the fire in the stomach. The 'jvarahari dravam' contained quinine, to cure a fever.

To this day, doctors trained in Ayurvedic medicine as well as modern western medicine are available for consultation at the Charitable Hospital in Kottakkal and there are two counters dispensing both kinds of medicine, keeping this tradition alive. Simple and essential surgical procedures are performed in the hospital as well. From its inception, large crowds of patients flocked to the hospital for free treatment and medicines.

The first floor of the hospital building had a wide open verandah running along the entire length in front. This led into a drawing room, and beyond were three large rooms. Once this bungalow was ready, P.S. Varier often came at night from the Arya Vaidya Sala to sleep upstairs, since it was cool and pleasant there because of the open verandah.

At the back of the bungalow, behind the dispensary, a flight of steps led down to a large open courtyard with a covered corridor running through its centre. At the end of the corridor were ten rooms, five on each side, for in-patients. On either side of the rooms were two residential wings. The bigger, two-storeyed one, with a kitchen attached to it, was used by the chief teacher at the Patasala. The other wing was also two-storeyed but smaller, and had a kitchen outside. This was used by the staff of the Patasala.

On the right wing were two extra rooms that were used for women patients. On the left were two kitchens, one for cooking food, the other for heating oils and medicines. The well was adjacent to the kitchens. There was a small building at the back of the bungalow with two or thee rooms, which was used as a mortuary.

The Patasala, which has now been turned into a ward for patients who suffer the effects of poisoning, was a large L-shaped hall at the side of the hospital.

When classes in the Patasala began to function, Varier felt

there was an acute need for textbooks on Anatomy and Physiology. He therefore began to translate Gray's *Anatomy*, the most well-known textbook of the time, from English and portions of these translations appeared in successive issues of the *Dhanvanthari* magazine. His ultimate objective was to do a full translation of this textbook in eight volumes, but he knew even this would not be enough and there was far more work to do. He felt strongly that the advantages available to students of western medicine had to be taken into consideration while planning a textbook for students of Ayurveda:

> It is no secret that all important concepts in English medicine are finally accepted only after many worthy doctors pass different kinds of examinations and a majority of them agree on these concepts. And that is not all. They hold discussions with the practitioners of every kind of vaidyam current in modern countries. Also, they have the facilities to obtain and dissect dead bodies in order to study them. Because of all this, what physicians trained in English medicine say at the moment is more worthy of belief than what indigenous physicians say, especially in the field of Anatomy. Those who say that Sushrutha's Anatomy is completely correct should look at the meaning of the sloka given below and judge its veracity:

> *Pundareekena sadrisham hridayam syadadhomukham*
> *Jagrathasthadvikasathi svapathascha nimeelathi*

> The meaning of this is: 'the heart is like a lotus, and hangs face downwards. When it is awake, it is fully opened; when asleep, it closes.' Now, if the heart is fully open and hangs down, even a small child will know that it cannot hold anything. Then how can it contain a fluid force like energy? How can it deal with

the flow of blood? It is very difficult to agree on such matters. There are so many contradictions like this.[13]

Varier's own aim was to write a book in which the concepts in Ayurveda would be placed alongside those in western medicine in a comparative study that would benefit students of Ayurveda. He decided to write a book called *Brihadchchareeram* on these lines in Sanskrit, so that it would be available to readers and students outside Kerala as well. The opening verse describes the objective of the book:

Nanathanthrani samveekshya
Pracheenani navani cha
Siddha prathyaksha yukthibhyam
Siddhanthothra vilikhyathe

(Having studied old and new shastrams attentively, I write these principles with the real knowledge I have gained.)

The book was planned in a hundred and eight chapters that would be divided into eight sections: Histology, Osteology, Syndesmology, Myology, Angiology, Neurology, Splanchnology and Physiology. By the time Varier completed the first thirty-two chapters in three sections, however, Kaviraj Mahamahopadhyaya Gananath Sen of Calcutta published his *Prathyakshashareeram*, a textbook in Sanskrit on the same subject. Varier thought his book would become redundant and abandoned it for the moment.

However, when Varier started to use Gananath Sen's book in the Patasala, he felt that it did not fulfil all the requirements of the students. He therefore decided to write a short textbook that would cover the essential aspects of Anatomy and Physiology and began work on this in June 1924. This textbook,

[13]Varier, P.S.: 'Jnangalude Abhipraayam' (Our Opinion), *Dhanvanthari*, 17 October 1913.

called the *Ashtangashareeram*, took him only fourteen months to write and was ready in 1925. Varier worked very hard to finish it quickly, writing for hours together every day. He explains in the preface that the aim of the book is to provide students with concepts from Ayurveda that can incorporate the elements of modern medicine, particularly those that can be adapted and applied to the practice of Ayurvedic medicine. Varier writes:

A thorough knowledge of the human body is the foundation for Ayurveda. Charaka says:

Sarvada sarvatha sarva
Shareeram veda yobhishak
Ayurvedam sakartsnyena
Veda lokasukhapradam

(He who knows the human body in its completeness at all times in all ways knows Ayurveda, which gives happiness to all people. And this is why I write this.)

But all competent Ayurvedic physicians of the present day are unanimously of the opinion that the existing Ayurvedic treatises are both deficient and defective in the treatment of this subject. It is not, therefore, necessary to dwell on that point here at any length. It must nevertheless be emphasized that the first duty of a physician who desires to renovate the Ayurvedic system is to improve the anatomical and physiological side of it. This book is a result of the efforts inspired by these ideas.

I have always held that a mere translation of some of the English works on Anatomy and Physiology will not satisfy these requirements. My idea was that these branches of knowledge as already dealt with in Ayurveda should be revised on the same lines and augmented by

the necessary modern knowledge without repugnance
to the Ayurvedic system.[14]

In order to help students memorize the text of this book,
Varier wrote it in verse and included illustrations and a
commentary to explain difficult verses. English equivalents to
the Sanskrit words in the verses were also given in this
commentary. Since there were no synonyms in Sanskrit for
many terms used in Anatomy and Physiology as they were
studied in western medicine, Varier invented his own terms in
many cases. The book received great praise at the sixteenth
annual conference of the Akhila Bharatha Vaidya Samiti held
in Jaipur in 1926. A special citation was sent to P.S.Varier by
the President of the Samiti, Pandit Madan Mohan Malaviya.

Varier invites readers, in the preface to *Ashtangashareeram*,
to point out any errors they may find in the text, so that he
could discuss such errors with his colleagues and correct them
in a later edition. He says candidly that a text of this nature,
being a venture of a new kind, was bound to have drawbacks
that he was anxious to rectify.

Meanwhile, the *Oushadha Nirmana Kramam*, the booklet
on Pharmacy that he had written in 1910 setting out the
formulations for the processing of Ayurvedic medicines, had
been in his sole possession all these years, and he had been
personally supervising the processing procedures in the Vaidya
Sala. Only the vaidyan who was in charge of these procedures
had a copy of the booklet. From time to time, Varier had made
additions and alterations that he found necessary. S.R. Iyer,
who came to the Patasala as a teacher and who later became
the factory manager and special officer, edited a revised version
of this booklet, which is consulted in the Arya Vaidya Sala

---

[14]P.S. Varier: Preface to *Ashtangashareeram. Souvenir of the
Vaidyaratnam P.S. Varier's Centenary Celebration*, 1969, p.23.

even now. Written in a very simple, lucid style, it first gives the name of the indigenous medicine and quotes the appropriate formulation for processing it from the original Sanskrit text from which it is taken, citing the relevant chapter and section. The Sanskrit verse is then explained in Malayalam: the list of ingredients is given, followed by the method of processing, including the timings for each stage. Lastly, instructions are given on how to preserve the medicine. The book comes a long way from the time when a guru would quote a verse without giving any indication of which text it was from, leaving it to the student to identify it and carry out the formulation it cited.

These were years of intense and tremendous activity for P.S. Varier. He worked from six-thirty in the morning to eight at night, breaking off only to eat now and then. Writing a textbook for his students, plays for the drama troupe, articles for the *Dhanvanthari* magazine; coaching and directing the actors and musicians and composing songs for them; attending to patients from far and near and dealing with their correspondence; supervising the administration of the Arya Vaidya Sala, the Charitable Hospital, the Patasala; planning and constructing a series of new buildings—his days were so full that he could barely find time to visit the variam. Kutty Varasyar and her son, P.V. Krishna Varier looked after family affairs. P.S. Varier often spent the night, especially when it was hot, in the cool room over the hospital, where a breeze blew in through the wide verandah and he felt rested, at peace after a busy day.

From 1920 to 1925, Varier worked as a director in the Nedungadi Bank, Kozhikode. He resigned his post when his own activities began to claim too much time.

The status of the school run for the girls of Kottakkal inside the kovilakam suddenly became precarious at this time and the building they occupied had to be vacated. There was no money for a new building, and it looked as if the school would have to be moved out of Kottakkal. An appeal was made to Varier and he promptly contributed five hundred rupees. The school was able to survive in Kottakkal, to the relief of the students and teachers.

Flashes of the quirky, almost childlike flamboyance P.S.Varier was to develop in choosing his personal possessions as he grew older began to touch his life at this period. He designed a table at which he could write standing, since he found this comfortable when he wrote plays and articles. This table occupied a central space in his big room above the medicine store, next to the Arya Vaidya Sala. He started to use a small lamp, fashionable and rare in those days, that his father, Rama Varier, had given him. Known as a 'spring-lamp', it had a candle that kept rising above the rim of its stand, activated by a spring underneath. He carried this lamp everywhere after dark. He designed a small strong room off his bedroom in the Arya Vaidya Sala, to keep his valuables safe. It had double doors with inset brass locks in both. One door has now been dismantled, the other is still intact.

A peacock appeared on the premises of the Arya Vaidya Sala, and a cage where it could rest; Varier could look down from the landing outside his bedroom into the cage. But the peacock ran freely around the grounds of the Vaidya Sala most of the time, with a deer to keep it company.

The land over which the factory and office buildings of the Arya Vaidya Sala now sprawl measures roughly two acres and was acquired piecemeal by Varier in the course of these crowded years. He put up each structure as the need arose, the requirements of the Arya Vaidya Sala and the drama troupe receiving equal attention. The old buildings have been preserved with remarkable care, though each of them is now used for a different purpose than the one it was designed for. Although most of the people who now work in this vast complex are aware that the rooms they move around in have a century-old history, not many can identify the exact spaces. Sri P. Raghava Varier, the present AGM, is one of the few in the family who can still point out each spot with loving accuracy and recreate the story of its past.[15]

Below Varier's large bedroom, which is now the main office, is a big hall (now the finance department) which was used to store and pack medicines. Medicines that were sent by rail to distant places were packed here into wooden boxes. On the second floor, above Varier's bedroom, is a big hall where the artists in the drama company used to work. Stretching large pieces of cloth over the floor, the chief artist, Achutha Menon, designed curtains and backdrops for the plays. The walls of this room used to be covered with the rough sketches the artists made. Outside this room, on the southern side, is a small balcony where the bell that marked time for the factory workers still hangs in the small belfry, though it is silent now. It was rung at 6.45 in the morning, so that the workers could assemble at 7.00 and again at 1.45 in the afternoon, so that they could assemble at 2.00 for work after lunch. It was also rung if there was an emergency of some kind.

The full-length portrait that Achutha Menon drew of P.S. Varier now hangs in Sri P. Raghava Varier's room in the administrative office, which used to be Varier's own bedroom.

A permanent hall was built in 1912 on the north-east of the building where Varier stayed, for the drama troupe to stage their plays. The hall, which could seat seven to eight hundred people, now serves as a store for the herbs and plants which are brought to the factory for the manufacture of medicines. It used to have three sections: the first class spectators sat right in

---

[15]I owe all the information on the old buildings in Kottakkal and a description of what they were originally used for to Sri. P. Raghava Varier.

front in chairs, the second also sat in less comfortable chairs behind them and right at the back, on a raised platform, were the floor seats, which were the cheapest. The green room was behind the stage.

Two extra kitchens were added on behind the Arya Vaidya Sala building, with eight large fireplaces, since the quantity of medicines being processed had increased. Women who attended the performances of the plays went into the hall through a long corridor that ran by the side of this block and led right up to the performance hall. Men entered directly from the street in front of the Vaidya Sala.

A two-storeyed house with three rooms on the ground floor and another three on the second, a kitchen and a veranda, was put up for Shoolapani Varier, the manager of the drama troupe and his assistants. Being on the northern side of the Vaidya Sala, it came to be known as the vadakke pura, the northern house. There used to be a fairly big, rocky hill behind this house, to the west of it, called the Kuttichathan Para, the Demon Rock, which was levelled later. Varier built two structures on the hill: a lavatory for himself and a storage room for the petrol (which he bought in two-gallon cans) for the new Dodge car he purchased around this time. A small shed was built in front of the dispensary, near the compounding room, for the car.

By the side of the peacock cage there was a room used by S. Raghunatha Iyer (known affectionately to everyone as Iyer Master) when he moved from the Patasala, where he had been working as a teacher, to the Arya Vaidya Sala as factory manager.

All these buildings have the sloping tiled roofs typical of Kerala and rough floors of red country tiles. Except for the elegant doors of the strong room, the construction in the Arya Vaidya Sala was mainly functional. It is the lines of the Arya Vaidya Chikitsasala, the gracious 'bungalow', with its soaring two-tiered tiled roof, its high portico with wide arches, its open veranda on the first floor, that foreshadow the amazing architect of Kailasamandiram, the house that was soon to be built for the family.

12

The Revolt of 1921

P.S. Varier became deeply involved in the incidents in Malabar that came to be called by different names: the Peasants' Revolt, the Mapilla Rebellion, the Ernad Riots. Kottakkal was seriously affected by these incidents because of its proximity to Tirurangadi, one of the centres of turmoil. Varier's own role in the long drawn out drama was touched by the personal magnetism, the charisma that had by then become a part of his forceful personality.

Thanks to the generous sense of vision that had prompted Varier to start building the Charitable Hospital complex at a time when he could ill afford it, large sections of the poorer population had found work on the site. This gesture, added to the concern he always had shown all his patients and employees, had won him the loyalty and affection of the villagers and was to safeguard him and the village of Kottakkal through a tumultuous period.

The Khilafat movement in India grew out of the sense of grievance that Muslims all over the world bore against Britain for their role in the war of 1914 to 1918 and the threat of

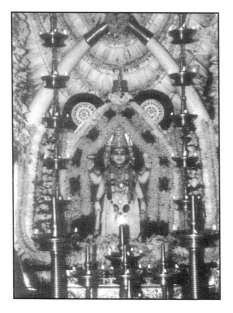

Vishvambharan, idol in Varier's temple

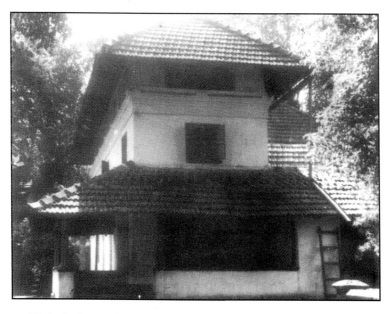

Varier's tharavad, or family house, where he spent his childhood

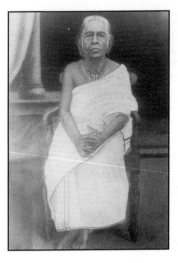

Ittichiri, Varier's Cheriyamma

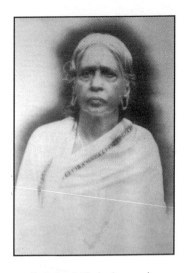

Lakshmi, Varier's cousin

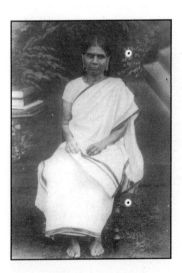

Kunji Varasiar (Parvathy),
Varier's cousin

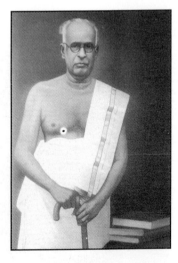

Kavikulaguru
P.V. Krishna Varier, Varier's
cousin

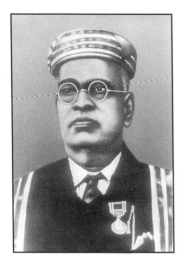

Varier, with the Vaidyaratnam title

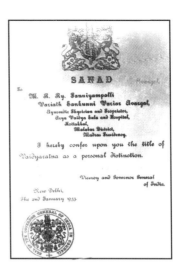

The Vaidyaratnam title

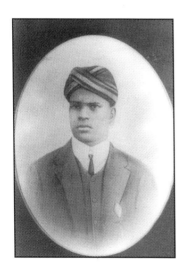

Varier, in his thirties

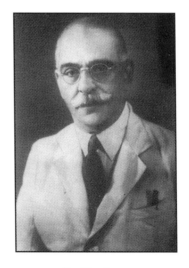

Dr Verghese

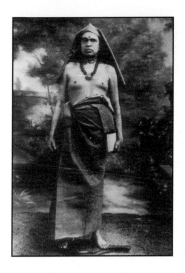 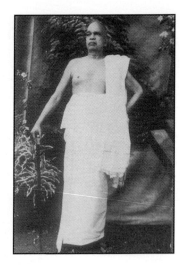

Varier, dressed in   Varier, in traditional Kerala
maravuri (bark)   costume

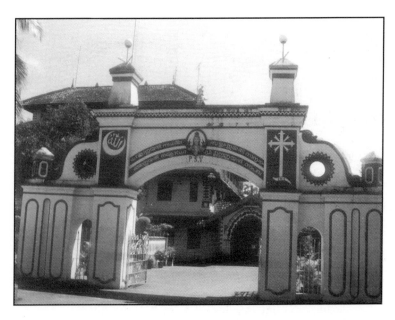

Gate of Kailasamandiram

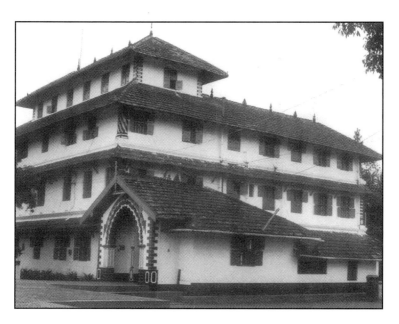

Kailasamandiram

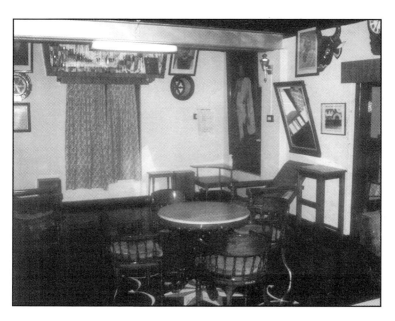

Varier's room, furnished according to his specifications

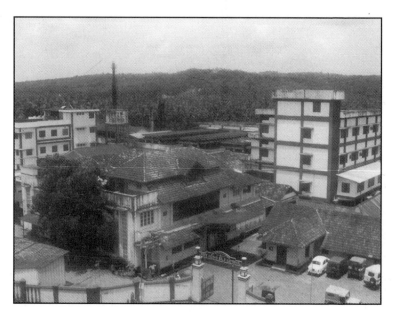

The Arya Vaidya Sala today

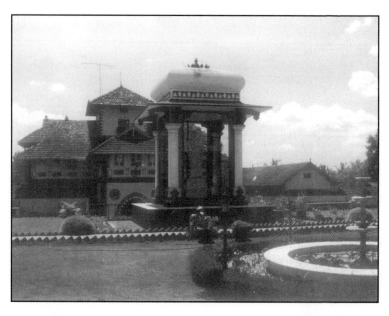

The Charitable Hospital

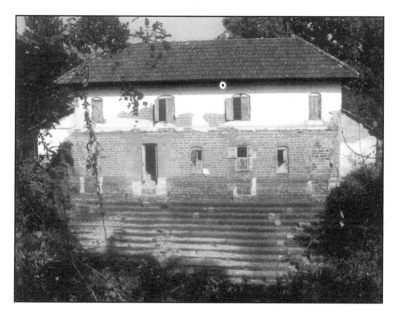

Kuttancheri Kulappura Malika, where Varier stayed as a student

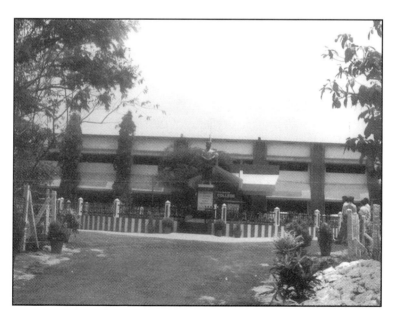

New premises of the Ayurveda College

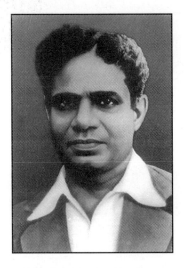

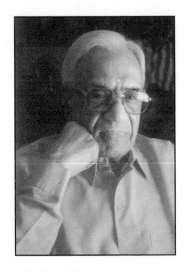

Dr P.M. Warrier, the first
managing trustee

Dr P.K. Warrier, the present
managing trustee

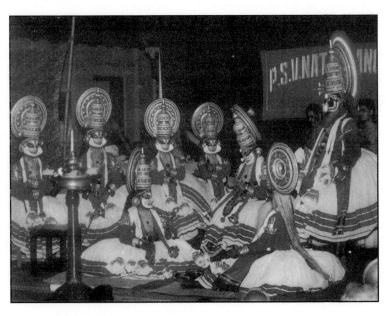

A scene from Kathakali performed by the PSV Natya Sangham

disintegration it posed to the Turkish Empire. The Mapilla Muslims of Malabar supported the Khilafat whole-heartedly and displayed their concern for the cause at the Congress conference held in Manjeri in 1920. The Khilafat workers decided to adopt the non-cooperation activities initiated by Gandhi to express their protest against Britain, thus allying themselves with the nationalist cause. In Kerala, particularly in Malabar, Congress and Khilafat committees worked in unison and the British authorities made every effort to suppress them.

In February 1921, when a group of Congress leaders comprising K. Madhava Menon, U. Gopala Menon and Ponmadath Moideen Koya prepared to welcome the Khilafat leader, Yakub Hassan, on his visit to Kozhikode, Hassan and the Congressmen were arrested. The next day, workers who belonged to both the Khilafat and Congress movements were arrested in the town of Tirurangadi and sentenced to six months' rigorous imprisonment. When they were released in August 1921, a reception was organized for them at the Parappanangadi railway station. They were to be met at the station and taken in procession to Tirurangadi, and the road was hung with festoons for the occasion. The British government forbade this reception and more than five hundred white policemen arrived in Tirurangadi on the night of 19 August under the leadership of the District Collector, Thomas and the District Superintendent of Police, Hitchcock. With the intention of arresting the Khilafat leader, Ali Musaliyar, they cordoned off the Khilafat office and mosque and made a search. They did not find Ali Musaliyar, but they did round up some other leaders. By dawn, the Mapillas who heard the news that the police had entered the mosque flocked to Tirurangadi from the surrounding areas. It was the day of the chanda, the weekly market, in Kottakkal. The Mapilla vendors abandoned their stalls to rush to Tirurangadi. They demanded the release of those who had been arrested. In answer, the British turned their guns on them. Seventeen Mapillas died, many were wounded. Four policemen were killed as well.

Riots directed against the government broke out in many places near Kottakkal: Ernad, Valluvanad, Ponnani, Kozhikode. Railway stations, offices and courts were attacked, treasuries were emptied. The rebels clashed with the British soldiers, there were many deaths. On 29 August, the Army surrounded the mosque in Tirurangadi, arrested Ali Musaliyar and many others. Ali Musaliyar and twelve others were hanged for treason.

For more than a year, the rioting continued and the British soldiers responded with continued atrocities. Unrest and terror spread through Malabar. To make matters worse, the riots suddenly turned against the wealthy Hindu landlords in Malabar. Many Hindus in Kottakkal fled to the royal family in the eastern kovilakam seeking refuge. A big group of Mapillas attacked the post office and the Registrar's office in Kottakkal, then gathered in the bazaar. Word reached P.S. Varier that they planned to attack the kovilakam next. Varier sent a messenger requesting the Mapilla leaders to come and meet him. Their chief set out at once, followed by his whole group. The people of the village drew back, terrified, certain that Varier's end had come.

Unruffled, Varier came out to meet the Mapillas. They told him they needed ·money desperately and asked for his support for their cause. He advised them to be careful: the British were powerful adversaries. He gave them money and reminded them gently that it was the Samoothiri rulers of Kozhikode who had first welcomed their forefathers to the Malabar shores. He requested them not to hurt anyone at the kovilakam and offered to send someone there to get them money for their cause, which he did forthwith. The Mapillas left, acknowledging him as a friend.

Many Hindus who felt threatened came from areas nearby

asking for shelter at the Vaidya Sala. Varier housed them in various buildings in the Arya Vaidya Sala compound and arranged for them to be fed. They brought their jewels and valuables to him for safekeeping. Among the refugees were the poorest of the poor and people from all castes. P.S. Varier, his cousin P.V. Krishna Varier and his niece's husband K.V. Sankara Varier talked to the Mapillas frequently, trying to dissuade them from hot-headed skirmishing and rioting.

Although most government activities came to a standstill for almost a year because of the climate of unrest and the continual breakout of riots, the business of the Arya Vaidya Sala was not interrupted. The Mapillas themselves regularly transported the raw materials P.S. Varier required for the manufacture of medicines to the Vaidya Sala. Varier's car was allowed to move in and out of Kottakkal freely. Indeed, letters and parcels were often taken in the car to Tirur and back, since postmen and messengers were afraid to carry them. Officials or women and children who were nervous about travelling to and fro were also transported in the car. The Arya Vaidya Sala workers were allowed to move around freely in the village as well.

Late one night, the post office authorities brought their money and records to the Vaidya Sala, asking Varier to look after them. Slowly, Muslim families who were afraid of the British soldiers began to find their way there as well, bringing their jewels, their pots and pans. No one was turned away. Varier gave them food and lodging and whatever other help he could until the organized teams of the Servants of India Society were able to take over from him and extend the necessary help to victims of the rioting.

A remarkable incident took place when G.K. Devadhar, the president of the Servants of India Society, visited Kottakkal. He offered P.S. Varier his congratulations on the measures he had taken to care for all those who had come to him for refuge. Varier took him completely by surprise when he told him that the Servants of India Society should not limit their relief measures to Hindus alone, they should extend them to Muslim women and children. But the Muslims are behind the riots, Devadhar countered, why should we help them? Varier answered that only men had taken part in the riots, that most of them had been arrested or fled the region and that, in either case, the women and children had been left helpless and starving. It was the first time in Malabar that Devadhar had heard someone argue for the Muslims. Moved by P.S. Varier's plea and respecting his large-heartedness, he reported the matter to the government and commented on it in an article he wrote for the *Times of India*, published from Bombay.

Varier wrote to the government himself and was able to obtain some help for the abandoned Mapilla families. When Sir Arthur Nape visited Kottakkal in connection with an enquiry the British were making into the riots, Varier reiterated his appeal on behalf of the Muslim women and children and Nape was as surprised as Devadhar had been.

Military rule was imposed in the region and policemen and soldiers flooded the streets. Unable and too impatient to distinguish rioters from the innocent, the police made countless arrests. Fortunately, the police officer who was in charge at Kottakkal was a relatively just and straightforward person. Since there were no convenient lodgings in the area, many of the police officers camped in the Arya Vaidya Sala buildings and P.S. Varier was for a while the protector of policemen, Hindu refugees and Mapilla refugees alike.

There is a family legend of how Varier defended a Mapilla bullock cart driver, Soopy, whom he had known for years and of whom he was very fond, against the British. The British police were combing the countryside and carrying off Mapillas by the hundreds. Soopy was in grave danger and came to Varier for help. Varier told him to stay in the Vaidya Sala and told the police that he had been there with him all the time and could not have been involved in the rioting. Soopy stayed there until the danger passed and he could come out safely.

Soopy did well for himself later in life, bought half an acre of land in Kottakkal and did not need to drive a bullock cart any more. It is said that he visited Varier every day after he retired from work, to pay him his respects.

Because of his impartial championship, Varier incurred the resentment of a section of the villagers who spread a rumour that he was a supporter of the Khilafat, that his cousin, P.V. Krishna Varier was a Khilafat man and that neither could be trusted. But Varier's actions had always been too open and straightforward to invite suspicion and the rumour died a natural death.

Resentment and jealousy are not always easy to quell, however, and there was a spate of anonymous letters to the kovilakam suggesting that P.S. Varier was an ally of the Mapillas and was working secretly against the kovilakam. The rumour mongers were not successful, but their efforts to provoke suspicion did irritate Varier.

Meanwhile, he had other things on his mind. K. Sankunni Varier, his able, trusted manager at the Kozhikode branch of the Vaidya Sala, caught smallpox and died within three days. He was a man with remarkable administrative skills and could have taken over from P.S. Varier at any moment, had he wished to hand over his responsibilities. His death was a great blow to Varier.

Members of the family kept falling ill as well, one by one, at the variam. Varier not only had a firm belief in astrology, he could cast and read horoscopes. He decided to have a prasnam done by one of the reputed astrologers of the time, Nalloor Gopala Panikker, to find out why the family was going through such a difficult phase. Gopala Panikker told him the omens were not good at all and even suggested that someone who bore Varier ill will was practising black magic against him. He advised him to have propitiatory rituals conducted. Varier's instinct was to disbelieve this. No black magic or illwill could hurt those who were honest and forthright, he declared. But within a month, he lost one of the most faithful workers in the factory, E. Sankunni Varier—he died of typhoid. Was it a coincidence, wondered P.S. Varier, that both the people who had died bore his name? Other workers fell ill. The employees of the Arya Vaidya Sala had come to know of the astrologer's advice and were unhappy that Varier had paid no heed to it. They seemed even more distraught than they had been at the time of the recent riots.

Varier was in a dilemma. He feared nothing for himself and felt he was answerable to no one since he believed there was no one in the world who would be directly affected by his death. If God so wished it, he would die; God would keep him alive if there was work for him to do. But the welfare of his workers was a different matter. He had always considered them, treated them, like his own children and he could not bear the thought that some misfortune might befall them because of his carelessness. He felt that people whom he had thought of as close to him were turning against him at this juncture. In the end, he gave in, ordered that the rituals be performed and sent for a team of Namboodiris to do them.

The section of villagers that was determined to bring about his downfall were meanwhile presented, quite by chance, with another opportunity to discredit him. They had already convinced Jamedar Kurup, one of the police officers of the Malabar Special Police (M.S.P.), who had been asked to camp in Kottakkal following the riots, that P.S. Varier and the Arya Vaidya Sala workers were arrogant and insufferable and needed to be taught a lesson. Kurup waited, biding his time. A man named Ayyappa Menon came from Thrissur to spend some time in Kottakkal and persuaded Varier's trusted head clerk,

Shinnan Menon, who had been with Varier from the time he began the Vaidya Sala, to let him stay at his house. Shinnan Menon discovered very soon that the newcomer was not pleasant or desirable company and ordered him to leave. An argument followed and the ordinarily quiet and gentle Shinnan Menon lost his temper, grabbed Ayyappa Menon's stick from his hand and hit him with it! All this took place in front of Jamedar Kurup's place.

Shinnan Menon told Varier what had happened. Varier told him he had been wrong to hit Ayyappa Menon but advised him to lie low and wait. Ayyappa Menon's allies tried to persuade Shinnan Menon to pay a hundred rupees and close the affair, but Shinnan Menon refused, on Varier's advice. Late one night, soon after Varier came back from his consultations at the Kozhikode Vaidya Sala, Jamedar Kurup arrived in uniform with two armed policemen to threaten Varier for not settling Shinnan Menon's case. 'Do you understand what military power is?' roared Kurup belligerently. 'How would I know what military power is?' retorted P.S. Varier, unperturbed, 'I know only the power of thiktham kashayam, a medicine I make here in my factory!' Kurup, who had been drinking, was infuriated and began to shout at Varier. The factory employees gathered outside, frightened, wondering what was going to happen.

Just then, Inspector Chummar, a police inspector who had arrived from British Cochin, walked in. Jamedar Kurup paled when he saw him. He had worked under the Inspector earlier. When Kurup had been dismissed from the department for various misdemeanours, it was Inspector Chummar who had taken pity on him and let him go without too severe a punishment. Kurup had then joined the Malabar Special Police. He was not at all happy to meet Chummar again, and in such embarrassing circumstances! Giving him a perfunctory salute, he left as quickly as he could.

The Inspector had come on an errand that Varier was well aware of. The villain of this whole episode, Ayyappa Menon, had been extracting money from a woman in Thrissur over many months, promising to get her daughter married to one of the young men at the Kottakkal kovilakam. Growing suspicious, the woman, who knew P.S. Varier, had requested him to find out what was going on and Chummar had actually been sent to Kottakkal to arrest the culprit. All that the unfortunate Jamedar Kurup got for his pains was to be dismissed from the M.S.P. as well for his most recent misbehaviour!

Over the years, Varier had found a steady and trusted friend in a man named Ambi Iyer, who was related to Shinnan Menon. Ambi Iyer belonged to an extremely poor family whose home was in the village of Koduvayur. His older brother had found work in the kovilakam at Kottakal and Ambi Iyer came to Kottakkal as a child, following his brother, hoping he could somehow earn his living there. Like many others in similar circumstances, he ate at the kovilakam, did odd jobs and bided his time, wondering how to find work. A chance came his way quite unexpectedly: during the monsoon one year, the kovilakam ran out of firewood and was in a desperate situation. Ambi Iyer offered to find a consignment of firewood somewhere and deliver it to them. He kept his word. The thampuran of the kovilakam was pleased and handed over the charge of the storeroom of the kovilakam to him, a heavy and profitable responsibility. Ambi Iyer put away the money he earned carefully. In seven years, he made seven thousand rupees, no mean capital. Ambi Iyer then established his own business. He began to lend money at interest. He also started a bus service between Kottakkal and Tirur.

Ambi Iyer had known Varier ever since he came to Kottakkal and they had gradually become good friends. Varier enjoyed his company and always invited him when he went to see his troupe perform a play. If he was late, Varier would send someone to fetch him. Ambi Iyer would sit down next to Varier and pronounce his unvarying opinion, 'Magnificent!' One of the reasons why Varier liked him so much was that he was one of the very few people he knew who never asked a favour for himself. Varier respected him deeply for this. Theirs was an easy and affectionate companionship, neither made demands on the other.

And so the year 1927 arrived, following a long period that had brought Varier many anxieties and much grief. This was a year that was to mark an important and happy milestone, the twenty-fifth year since the Arya Vaidya Sala came into existence.

The year of the Silver Jubilee of the Arya Vaidya Sala was also the year when Varier began to write his diaries. The first entry on the first of January 1927.

1 January

Temperature 79° Pulse—lying down: 74. Seated—78. Standing—84. Urine 1016°. Body weight: after a motion, before coffee, with bare skin, wearing only a kaupeenam, 176 pounds. It is very cloudy. Kottur Raman has gone to Mannazhi, will not come today. Pulse at 9.15, seated in the easy chair—92. Respiration: 19. Pulse, standing—110, respiration: 22-23.

Went to the hospital. Raghava Varier, Madhavan Nair, Nedungadi were there. Lots of patients. At 2 p.m., inside heat 82. At 3.30, outside temperature 90°. Evening, specific gravity of urine 1020°.

The bustle and noise in the compound of the Arya Vaidya Sala had been growing steadily over these years. Many more workers reported to the processing section (which was by now known as the factory) than twenty-five years ago. The members of the drama troupe had their living quarters in the same compound and made their own contribution to the liveliness of the atmosphere. And since the performance hall was also in this compound, the evenings brought crowds of spectators from outside. As a consequence of all this, Varier no longer felt as comfortable as he used to in the room above the medicine store. He hardly saw the women and children of the family, since he seldom had time to visit the variam. Why not, he thought, construct a new house where the whole family could stay, where he would have his own space—a house where he could invite visitors, relax, join the family for meals. The idea took root within his restless, active, fertile mind. He had been building a great deal over the last few years and had learnt much about plans, building materials, methods of construction. This would be the most carefully thought out, the most ambitious structure . . .

The diary entries in 1927 are full of plans for this new residence. Konath Sankara Varier, a scholar of the science of building, helped P.S. Varier with the engineering aspects.

6 January 1927

Konath Sankara Varier came . . . He said the centre of the compound must be left empty and that it is better to dig the well on the eastern side. If there are 12 rings of 36 cm, the central soothram (of the house) will not clash with the middle point of the well, he said.

The 'soothram' provides cross ventilation and consists of small apertures placed along a continuous line in the walls of a house. It includes the openings—doors, windows, courtyards— along its course. Even if all the windows and doors in the house are closed, the soothram ensures air circulation.

19 April 1927

6 a.m. Temperature 86°. Pulse, seated: 81. Urine specific gravity 1020° . . .

Wrote to Kozhikode and Palakkad for iron beams. From the day before yesterday, the bathing tank on

the north is being emptied. The work is not over.
Musaliyar came in the evening. Looked at the work.
Spoke about the money. The vaastu bali has been fixed
for Friday.

Tea at 3.30. With slices of tender coconut. Tamarind
curry at night. Went to Edarikode.

29 July 1927

Decided the wall of the southern hall would be 12
threads (36 mm) thick. And the western wall of the
kitchen would be 12½ (54 mm).

Varier records having the vaastu bali performed according to
tradition on 22 April 1927. This is a ritual to invoke a blessing
on the land on which the house would be built and to dispel
any evil omens that might affect it. He also notes the amounts
of the dakshina paid to the priests.

While the big family house was being built, Varier's
concern for the buildings in the Arya Vaidya Sala continued:

11 August

... Am wondering whether to extend the drama hall
eastwards.

17 August

... The wood brought the day before yesterday is not
quite wide enough. Is only 13½. Stumps were fixed to
start the work of extending the drama hall eastward.

This was the year that young A.C. Achuthan first came to
Kottakkal for treatment. P.S. Varier records his arrival:

2 June 1927

... A.C.Achuthan came with his uncle. The uncle
went back in the afternoon. Went to the hospital in
the evening as well because Reddy needed to see me.

Made Achuthan sing at dusk. He finds it difficult to go
up a high register. I think his voice changes when he
does so . . .

The Dodge car he had bought at this time was clearly a
possession Varier delighted in, although Gopalan Nair, the first
chauffeur appointed to drive this car, proved an unfortunate
choice. Varier had taken the trouble to send him to Madras to
learn driving when he bought the Dodge. But Gopalan Nair's
addiction to alcohol made him unreliable at the wheel. Varier
hated the idea of dismissing a worker, so he had to think of a
way to keep him employed. He finally decided to buy another
car for himself, for which he appointed a new chauffeur,
Narayanan. He then sent the Dodge and Gopalan Nair to
Shoolapani Varier, explaining to him that he was sure to find
the car useful when distributing notices for the performances
and the like. The gentle Shoolapani Varier somehow put up
with this unhappy situation for a year although he was
continually harassed by the brawls and arguments that Gopalan
Nair got into. At the end of the year, Shoolapani Varier went
to P.S. Varier in despair. He said he would rather manage
without a car than endure Gopalan Nair any longer! Varier
was in a dilemma again. Unwilling to dismiss the driver
summarily, he gifted the car to him, telling him to run it as a
taxi and earn his livelihood. Gopalan Nair sold the car within
the year, for the handsome sum of eighty rupees, to buy
himself drink! In course of time, he arrived sick and helpless in
the Charitable Hospital, where he met his end.

Varier hated having to dismiss any of his workers and
always worried about their future careers if they did go away.
For instance, when one of the harmonium players in the
drama troupe insisted on leaving, Varier bought him a
harmonium, so that the man would not find it difficult to earn
a living on his own. The poor man did not make a success of
his life though, and not only sold the harmonium but was

obliged to return, chastened, to Kottakkal, where Varier unhesitatingly took him back into service.

Narayanan, the chauffeur who succeeded Gopalan Nair, was not very good at his work, but at least he remained sober. Varier often refers to the maintenance of the car in his diaries:

16 June

... Narayanan sent by the Mail to Coimbatore to have the battery of the car repaired.

17 June

Narayanan has come back. The battery will be ready on Tuesday.

24 June

The car is all right ... When going to the hospital at night, there was a cow on the road. The car swerved and fell into a ditch and the bumper is damaged.

Varier makes frequent references in his diaries to his outings in the car in the evenings, short drives with his companions to neighbouring villages which he obviously enjoyed. He also used the car to make his weekly visits to Kozhikode where he saw patients at the Vaidya Sala.

13

The Arya Vaidya Sala Silver Jubilee

The Silver Jubilee of the Arya Vaidya Sala was celebrated on 16 October 1927. It was a splendid event, in which the entire population of Kottakkal took part. The village was transformed: all the streets and shops were hung with festoons and towards evening, it was illuminated with thousands of lamps. There was a feast to which everyone was invited and a play was staged that evening without tickets for whoever wanted to see it. Offerings were made in all the temples and mosques in the vicinity. A reception was arranged for P.S. Varier to which people were invited from all over Kerala. Letters and telegrams poured in from those who could not attend the function.

Photographs were taken of all the employees of the Arya Vaidya Sala and the Charitable Hospital and of the students and teachers of the Patasala.

At the meeting in the evening, Varier read a report[16] of all the activities of the Arya Vaidya Sala, the Patasala and the

---

[16]Report read by P.S. Varier at the Silver Jubilee of the Arya Vaidya Sala, *Shashti Varshika Charithram* (A History of Sixty Years) published by E.P. Krishna Varier, Norman Printing Bureau, Calicut, 1929.

Chikitsasala. He also gave an account of the textbook he had written, the *Ashtangashareeram*, and of the drama troupe. He concluded the report with his hopes for the future.

Speaking about the Arya Vaidya Sala, he said with justifiable pride that he had not been obliged to close it for even a day although they had passed through troubled times (the World War, the Mapilla Riots, the floods of 1924) in the twenty-five years that had gone by. He described the period in which it had been established:

> Although there were some excellent vaidyans at the time, because of the difficulties in procuring medicines and because vaidyans themselves did not take up this responsibility, the majority of the educated employed and the rich had begun to seek the help of doctors trained in western medicine. Even the few exceptions there were had an inclination to turn in that direction. But their state of mind has gradually changed since the establishment of the Arya Vaidya Sala. If not the majority, at least a significant number have come back to Ayurveda with greater faith than before.

P.S. Varier spoke of how he had started the Arya Vaidya Sala with a modest capital that he had earned himself as a vaidyan; of how neither the people of the village nor the people in his own family had thought he would make a success of it. He then cited figures:

> In the first year medicines worth only Rs 1033 were sold in the Arya Vaidya Sala. But we made gradual progress and the sum rose to Rs 10,215 in the fifth year, Rs 28,936 in the tenth year, Rs 45,857 in the fifteenth year and Rs 71,052 in the twentieth year ... Speaking of the twenty-fifth year—that is, until September 1927—the figure from the sale of medicines has gone up to Rs 97,689. Rs 22,885 of this is from Kozhikode, Rs 9256 from Kottakkal and the remaining

Rs 65,548 from parcels sent by post and rail to distant
places . . . This year we have treated 16,017 patients in
the Vaidya Sala, 22,162 in the Charitable Hospital and
4,272 in the Kozhikode branch, making a total of
42,451 patients. (This does not include patients treated
through correspondence).

Speaking of the drama troupe, he set out the reasons for his
having become involved in such a venture:

1. The Arya Vaidya Sala employees do not have as
   many opportunities to find work in summer as they
   do in the rainy season, since they cannot pluck any
   medicines then. Therefore, other work must be
   found for them in those periods.

2. If a profit is made, it can be used for the growth of
   the Charitable Hospital.

3. All large establishments should have arrangements
   for entertainment.

4. Many more people can be given employment in the
   name of this company.

5. It would be an added advantage if this venture is
   able to dissuade people from other states putting on
   plays of an improper nature and grabbing money in
   this way.

6. If, thanks to this, good plays can be put on in the
   language of Kerala, they will be an embellishment
   to the literature of Kerala.

He talked of how twenty-four plays had been translated into
Malayalam and how a certain number of Tamil plays had been
left untranslated because they were useful to have in the
repertoire if the troupe went outside Kerala. He invited the
audience to judge for itself from that evening's performance

how much progress the troupe had made in all aspects of theatre: acting, music, stage props.

The final section of the report was a forerunner of the remarkable will Varier wrote before his death, a testimony to his constant wish that his endeavours should be carried on by his successors with no detriment whatsoever to the cause to which he had dedicated himself:

THE FUTURE

Since the Arya Vaidya Sala has been established and is being run by one person, I understand that many people are anxious about what might happen in the absence of that person. But I do not have any such anxiety. For I have never been arrogant enough to think at any time that I achieved all this by my own strength. It was God's wish that the decline of Ayurveda be stopped and that systematic progress be made in the process of its revival. All I feel is that He decided that I too was to be a humble contributor among the many who were to carry out that command. I am certain God would have found a way to maintain this progress. Still, human endeavour is also necessary here. '*Daive niveshya kuru paurushamatmashakthya*' (calling upon God, do your duty according to your capacity) goes the saying. Therefore, I consider it my duty to make certain arrangements to enable us to continue as we have been doing. What I want to do is register the Arya Vaidya Sala as a charitable establishment with certain stipulations and be able to hand over its administration before I retire to a committee which possesses the will and capacity to run it and make it function according to my objectives and ideals.

Varier astonished his workers by giving each of them a bonus in keeping with his post. It was not a concept they knew much about—but was certainly one that gave them great pleasure!

Mangalapatrams congratulating P.S. Varier on his achievements and wishing him continued success were presented to him by the people of Kottakkal, by all the employees in his establishments and by the Mapillas of Kottakkal. Among the many good things his employees thanked him for, they particularly mentioned his reluctance to dismiss workers:

> We believe that it will not be arrogance on our part to say that we have a right to be particularly satisfied that the Arya Vaidya Sala has become so prosperous. We would like to tell you that each of us does the work we have been allotted with the utmost pleasure and satisfaction, under your supervision and in accordance with your valued counsel. Each of us considers it his great good fortune to get a post of some kind in the Arya Vaidya Sala or in the establishments connected with it. Apart from the fact that every employee is given many facilities, there is another most important factor: that it is your firm decision that unless a person leaves for some serious reason, you will not, as far as possible, dismiss anyone. It is because you have always forgiven our mistakes with kindness, encouraged each of us in our specific work and bent the rules to help us in every way that we are able to do our appointed tasks.

The mangalapatram presented by the Mapillas of Kottakkal was inspired by deep emotion:

> . . . It was after the thampurans of the eastern kovilakam settled down permanently here that this region, which had been completely rustic until then, earned fame and importance. Manorama Thambatti's name and that of her son, Shaktan Samoothiripad Thampuran, who died in 1856, will never be forgotten in the history of the

Kottakkal region. And it is well known that it is thanks to the Eralpad Thampuran who died in 1879 that many modern features came to Kottakkal and that we, the Mapillas, were given numerous facilities for trade in this place ... Everyone will accept the fact that apart from the efforts of our thampurans, it is mainly the Arya Vaidya Sala that is behind the name and fame of the Kottakkal region. In the twenty-five years since the Arya Vaidya Sala was established, it is hard to describe the different kinds of help it has extended to humble people like us. The number of destitute patients among the Mapillas who have been saved by the Vaidya Sala is endless ... From the time the Arya Vaidya Sala was established, jobs of all kinds have increased in number, in proportion to the progress made each year. Since most of these jobs are done by our people, many of us have found a means of livelihood here. In short, if our growing population is taken into consideration, it is certain that it is because of this establishment, the Arya Vaidya Sala, that many of the poor among us are able to earn their livelihoods without leaving this village ...

... You have made your magnanimity in the religious affairs of us Mapillas clear in many ways. We believe that if all those prominent citizens who make speeches saying that Hindus and Mohammedans should unite and work together would only follow your footsteps, there would be a lasting friendship between Hindus and Muslims in this country.

After the reading of the mangalapatrams a huge procession of people set out from the Vaidya Sala, followed by a group of Mapillas performing kolkali, in which the dancers keep time tapping sticks against each other. Some of Kottakkal's prominent

citizens came next, accompanied by a band. Then came three
caparisoned elephants, the one in the middle carrying a statue
of Dhanvanthari. They were accompanied by drummers and
followed by yet another crowd of people. This long procession
wound its way through the decorated streets to the Charitable
Hospital. Halting there for some time, they were joined by
men carrying gaslights and flaming palm-leaf torches. They
started out again, went back the way they had come, passed the
Arya Vaidya Sala and stopped at the gate to the kovilakam by
eight at night. It was the first procession of its kind to be held
in Kottakkal and a memorable one: nothing as splendid and
elaborate had ever been seen in those parts before.

At eight-thirty, there was a feast for everyone. The play
began at nine. The company had chosen *Valliammal Charithram*
(The story of Valli), a play that could demonstrate the talents
of the actors and the excellence of the props very well. There
was tremendous applause when the six-headed Lord
Subramanian appeared to his devotees on top of a hill. There
was a huge audience since no one had to buy tickets; people
had come and taken their places hours ahead of time.

The *Malayala Manorama* of 22 October, the *Keralapatrika*
of 22 October, the *Mathrubhumi* of 5 November and the
Pratidinam of 25 October made special mention of the event.

The tremendous enthusiasm with which the residents of
Kottakkal participated in the Silver Jubilee celebrations was
eloquent proof of their appreciation for Varier and the work
he was doing. The Arya Vaidya Sala was by now well known
not only in Kerala but all over south India and in the north as
well.

The Arya Vaidya Sala owed a great part of its success to
the kind of meticulous attention Varier paid to its every
aspect—the purity of the ingredients used to process medicines,
the correctness of the consistencies they had to arrive at, the
compactness with which they were sealed and packed. Apart

from attending to the most minute of these details, Varier's vigilance reached out to the personal lives of his workers, to the needs of their families, the welfare of their children.

The organized system of correspondence that Varier had insisted the Vaidya Sala should maintain regularly helped him to be in contact with patients in the most distant places. The letters that poured in were first copied out in a register[17] and assigned reference numbers. They were not necessarily copied in full: information that was irrelevant was omitted by whoever went through them and the contents of each letter were accordingly abridged. Varier spent one or two hours every day going through this register, making a diagnosis on the basis of the information the letters gave and dictating replies in which he conveyed his comments and advice to the patients. These replies were then copied out neatly and sent back along with whatever medicines Varier had prescribed. This meant that there had been a fair amount of clerical work at the Arya Vaidya Sala from the time of its inception. This was one of the reasons why Varier always insisted on his staff being literate. Once they had learnt their letters, he personally supervised them to make sure they wrote as legibly and as elegantly as possible.

The colours and sounds of the Silver Jubilee celebrations still filled the air as the last spectator left the hall after the play. Varier was aware of a feeling of deep contentment: the Vaidya Sala had lived up to its promise; from the Patasala he had waited for for so long would soon emerge a new generation of vaidyans. One of them, he knew, would have to take over the work that he had only begun. The last few years had shown

---

[17]This information was furnished by A.C. Achuthan Nair, who performed this duty for many years.

him who it might be: eighteen-year-old Madhavan, his aunt Kutty Varasyar's grandson, who had enrolled in the Patasala two years ago, seemed a logical choice. Frail and inclined to bouts of ill-health, but with a mind whose brightness never failed to astonish and delight. Varier loved to teach the boy, provoke his agile intelligence to ask searching questions, watch the answers flash radiantly in his eyes ...

14

Kailasamandiram Takes Shape

A number of people, including his Cheriyamma, Kutty Varasyar, tried to discourage Varier from building the new house on the land he had bought next to the Vaidya Sala. A diary entry on 3 September 1927 records Kutty Varasyar's disapproval:

3 September

Went to the variam in the evening. Came back feeling distressed because Cheriyamma spoke disparagingly about the construction of the new house.

It was rumoured that inauspicious objects had been found in the soil at the site for the new building and that the omens were not good. 'We can make it a good place,' was Varier's unvarying answer to all the adverse comments. After the vaastu bali, the blessing invoked on the land, he performed all the propitiatory rites that he had been advised to do before he started building the house. One of the instructions the priests gave him that day was that he should always serve food to all who came to the house he was going to build. This remains a rule even now: no one who visits goes away without having a meal.

The house constructed by Varier is called Kailasamandiram and is built in the traditional Kerala style with two open courtyards or nadumuttams flanked by pillars as their pivotal points. It has four storeys and a sloping tiled roof. Its total plinth area is 15,661 square feet.

The large brass-studded door on the south-west, a traditional point of entry for Kerala houses, opens from the covered portico at the entrance into a formal sitting room. A staircase at the southern corner of this room goes up to Varier's private suite on the first floor. The ceiling of the sitting room is supported by steel girders branching out from a pillar placed near the door, a massive pillar with a girder embedded inside it. There is a small room on the north-west side of the sitting room.

Entering the inner portion of the house through the drawing room, a corridor leads northward to a staircase to the first floor. Along this corridor are two rooms, the machu (a room entirely panelled in wood, originally used as a granary) and the northern room, the vadakke ara, which is mainly used by the women of the house.

As one walks eastward through the door from the sitting room the main courtyard, the nadumuttam, is on the left, with a tulasi platform in the middle of it. On the right of the verandah running along the open side of the nadumuttam is the thekkini thara, the southern section with a raised platform, the most spectacular section of the house. Along the adjacent verandah on the eastern side of the courtyard is a smaller platform. About eighty leaves can be laid at a time for a meal on both the platforms together. The platform on the south, the larger one, has a magnificent jackwood beam running across its length to support the roof. It is a single piece, thirty-eight feet long, fifteen inches wide and eleven inches thick and was transported from Vengara laid on two bullock carts. The story goes that the officer who examined it at the checkpost when it was brought past Vengara was so amazed at its gigantic proportions that he made enquiries, found out for whom it was and visited the house to see how it had been used! Holding up this beam are three pillars of finely dressed black stone, one of which has the carving of a serpent on it. A staircase on the south-east end of this platform leads to the suites upstairs.

Beyond the main courtyard of the southern section is the dining room for the family, with a large kitchen adjacent to it, on the east. The storeroom is on the western side. The outer door of the dining room leads to the northern wing, where there is another, smaller courtyard. Beyond it is a big hall and two kitchens, a storeroom, rooms for the servants and a loft for stacking firewood. One of the small kitchens here is used mainly for warming oils for treatment. Off the hall of the northern wing, on the western side, is a room women use at delivery time.

Once the house was ready, all the members of the drama troupe ate together in the northern wing, seated on the wide verandas around its courtyard. Women seldom entered this portion of the house, since it was always filled with noisy men, their laughter and chatter.

The staircase from the sitting room leads directly into P.S. Varier's suite on the first floor. The rails of this staircase have hinges about two feet from the top and this section of each rail can be folded upwards. The doors above the staircase can then be closed and locked so that no one can go up. This ensured Varier privacy once he went upstairs to rest, and personal safety in times of turmoil.

The stairs terminate in a small landing which opens into Varier's elegant sitting room, which doubles now as a conference hall. Furniture was ordered for this room from Spencer and Company, Madras. There are four large upholstered rosewood easy-chairs and a small, circular marble-topped table with a single leg of carved rosewood. There are four ordinary upholstered chairs as well. The floor is black with criss-cross lines and the section under the table has a white and red pattern. Four framed Belgian mirrors are hung on the northern and southern walls. Two circular decorative ventilators with green glass panes are set in the eastern wall and two on the western wall. The windows also have panes of green glass, probably to temper the glare of the sunlight, which Varier always found difficult to bear because of his eye ailment.

Two long glass showcases at either end of the room, fixed to the wall, hold some of the gifts Varier received for his sixtieth birthday.

There are two bedrooms on either side of this sitting room. The one on the south has a small anteroom where Varier used to light a lamp and do his meditation and prayers. This is the room in which he died. He lighted the lamp here morning and evening. In the morning, it was a traditional Kerala nilavilakku, a long-stemmed oil lamp made of bell metal; in the evening, it was Varier's 'spring lamp' with the candle. This anteroom has a big window on the east opening on to a verandah. This is where the children of the family used to gather and wait for their valia ammaman, their great-uncle, to throw them sweets, usually pastel-coloured peppermints ordered from Madras, through the window.

The bedroom on the north still has the original cot with a brass bedhead, another item of furniture that Varier bought from Spencer and Company, Madras. The anteroom opens into the strong room where Varier kept his cash and valuables. It has double doors of polished wood fitted with brass locks. The one on the inner door chimes when it is locked or unlocked. The strong room has panelled walls of polished teak wood and double windows, both of which are fitted with bars.

On the other side of this bedroom is a room Varier

designed for Ayurvedic treatment, with ample space on the floor for the long wooden plank (the droni) on which the treatment is done. It opens into a bathroom on the northern side. Medicated water to be used for a bath after a session of treatment can be brought to this bathroom through a staircase leading from the kitchen area. Adjacent to this bathroom and next to the staircase is a suite of rooms in which A.C. Achuthan Nair, the actor-turned-vaidyan, stayed for many years. A staircase on the northern side of the house leads directly from outside to this suite. The bedroom on the north opens on the eastern side onto a landing from which a staircase goes down to the kitchen area. Varier usually ate his lunch and dinner on this landing. Seated on the floor, he ate off a banana leaf, facing east for lunch and west for dinner. His cousin Lakshmi Varasyar, Kutty Varasyar's daughter, a beloved childhood playmate, used to keep him company while he ate. Kottur Raman Varier, his cook from the time he moved to the room over the Vaidya Sala, brought the food by the kitchen staircase and served him.

Along the veranda where the children used to gather to ask for sweets are three independent rooms. The veranda looks down into the courtyard downstairs. There are three main staircases leading to the first floor from different points, ensuring the privacy of each suite.

All the floors in the house are the traditional polished black floors of Kerala. The woodwork is rich and solid.

There are three independent suites on the second floor with their own verandas. Each suite has a bedroom, a sitting room, a toilet and dressing room. The third floor, which is traditionally a thattin-puram, a small space directly below the tiled roof generally used for storage, is raised to this level only on the western side of the house. It consists of three big halls with high ceilings. The large windows in the halls look out on a marvellous view of Kottakkal. These rooms are spacious enough to be converted any time into a single suite or a set of independent rooms.

Although the house has all the features of a traditional Kerala taravad house built strictly according to the principles of vaastu, it has distinctive features envisaged by a mind that had acutely observed the shortcomings of the traditional style and wished to modify them. The ceilings are much higher than in the old Kerala houses and the windows larger, designed to let in as much light and air as possible, in sharp contrast to the small, dark rooms that are common in older houses. Particular care has been paid to ventilation—even when walking through the maze of rooms within the house there is a sense of light pouring in from outside, a feeling of unrestricted space, an awareness of loving, considered attention to detail.

There is evidence everywhere in the house of an agile mind at work, of a vision and imagination that has used a whole wealth of experience to make every detail as elegant and beautiful as possible, discarding anything dingy, narrow or ugly.

When he occupied Kailasamandiram, which he thought of as the puthen variam, the new variam (and this is how he refers to it in his diaries), Varier entered a new phase of life. After years of living by himself in the Vaidya Sala, he became a family man again. He ate with the family on special occasions, on birthdays and festival days, he became a loved and loving avuncular figure to the children of the household, his presence and authority were impressed on the rhythms of the household. He followed a disciplined routine: regular mealtimes, simple food, times set apart for prayer and work. But he took delight in his outings in the car with all the small children in the house, in his long evening walks with friends, in entertaining visitors, in his growing connections with the outside world.

It is certain that he must have gone carefully through catalogues in order to choose the kind of furniture he had sent from Madras. He used to have Spencer's soda sent as well and biscuits—cream crackers and Nice biscuits—articles of food that would certainly not have been available in small villages like Kottakkal at that time. He alludes frequently in his diaries to having eaten these with his evening tea.

By this time he had also adopted a style of dress that combined the traditional and the modern. Over his pristine white mundu, he wore a shirt, a tie and a black coat. On his head, he wore either a black felt cap or a ready-made turban. Many photographs show a long gold bordered angavastram, folded narrow and looped around his neck. He had a pocket watch and carried a walking stick as he grew older. He sometimes wore shoes and socks with this attire.

He worked no less hard in these years, nor did he slow down in any way in the meticulous attention he paid to all his establishments and their day-to-day administration. Nevertheless, he had grown into a social figure, a citizen of substance, a man who had learnt how to spend money with elegance, who was neither extravagant nor mean.

P.S. Varier wanted to have Kailasamandiram ready in time for his sixtieth birthday in April 1929, so that the birthday celebrations could coincide with the grihapravesham, the house-warming ceremonies. The construction progressed steadily under his constant supervision.

Destiny had always held grief in store for him and this period was no exception. On 17 May, 1928, he lost a valuable member of the drama troupe, a young man named C.P. Kuttikrishna Menon, an expert at playing women's roles and an excellent singer. He had been with the Parama Shiva Vilasam troupe for twelve years. Two years after he joined them, he had developed tuberculosis. Varier had always treated him with particular care because of his ill health and had arranged for surgery to be performed on him three times. While rehearsing the *Krishna Leela* that year, the actor fell seriously ill and did not improve even though Varier lavished attention on him. His death devastated Varier.

But more was to follow. A contemporary of P.S. Varier's, Indyannoor Krishna Pisharoty, who had spent long periods in Varier's home and in the Vaidya Sala, died on 30 May 1928. Yet another person who was close to Varier died that year, in July—his father's nephew, Achutha Varier.

Meanwhile, the construction of the house progressed and the inflow of money from the Arya Vaidya Sala was better than ever before. Quite fortuitously, the grihapravesham ceremony Varier had planned for the new residence assumed an unexpected role. P.V. Krishna Varier asked P.S. Varier whether he could arrange for an important literary event, the third annual meeting of the Samastha Kerala Sahitya Parishad, to be held in Kottakkal in December 1928. P.S. Varier thought this a good idea and promised to extend all the help he could. As the time for the conference drew near, P.V. Krishna Varier told his cousin that it was proving difficult to arrange accommodation for all the invitees in Kottakkal. The new house was only half finished, but it had been fully tiled and P.S. Varier suggested at once that they suspend the construction and concentrate on making the completed portions habitable, so that they could be used for the literary conference.

Many people, including good friends of Varier and his relatives, were shocked when they heard of this plan. They thought it was not fitting to allow a big group of utter strangers belonging to different castes and creeds the use of a house which had not even been formally blessed according to traditional rites. True to his inclination for the unconventional, Varier was not deterred. It seemed to him most gratifying that a host of literary luminaries should be the first to move around his new house.

The twenty-ninth and thirtieth of December 1928 witnessed one of the most colourful events held in Kottakkal. K. Kunhunni

Varier, a Sanskrit scholar and poet, describes the reaction of the participants: when they reached Kottakkal, he said, they felt like Kuchelan, Krishna's old childhood friend, when he came upon Dwaraka, the abode of Lord Krishna. On the east of the road where the invitees arrived were the Arya Vaidya Sala, the drama hall, the kitchens for the preparation of medicines and next to them, the half-finished edifice of Kailasamandiram, where they were going to stay, looking like a marvel.

K.C. Veerarayan Raja of the royal Samoothiri family of Kozhikode gave the speech of welcome. He spoke of how Kottakkal had first made a name for itself in Malabar because of Manorama Thambatti whose erudition and gracious hospitality had drawn scholars from all over Kerala and as far away as the Chola region to visit Kottakkal. Over the last twenty-five years, however, he said that Kottakkal owed its great reputation to P.S. Varier's Arya Vaidya Sala. Apart from this, the two magazines, the *Dhanvanthari*, edited by P.S. Varier and the *Kavanakaumudi*, edited by his cousin P.V. Krishna Varier were both well known and appreciated in the literary world.

There were four sessions in all: on the first day, 29 December, proceedings began at 11 a.m., continuing up to 2 p.m. and from 3 p.m. to 6 p.m. On 30 December, the morning session was from 11 to 2 and the valedictory session from 3.00 to 8.00 in the evening. A young man in his twenties, G. Sankara Kurup, later to become one of Kerala's most renowned poets and the winner of the first Gnanapith Award, recited a poem he had written for the occasion. There were speeches by Punnassery Nambi Neelakanta Sharma of the Sanskrit College in Pattambi and the poet and historian, Ulloor S. Parameswara Iyer. Many leading literary figures of the day spoke at the sessions on the first day, including Attoor Krishna Pisharoty who had translated Kalidasa's *Shakunthalam* into Malayalam.

The morning session on 30 December was devoted entirely to women. B. Kalyani Amma, the writer and teacher who presided over the session, said in her speech that it was the first time a session had been set aside like this for women. The poets Kadathanattu K. Madhavi Amma, Thottekkatu Madhavi Amma, Tharavathu Ammalu Amma, Ambady Ikkavamma and Thottekkatu Gowri Kettilamma were present and their photographs appear in the volume commemorating the event. Many more poets and writers spoke at the valedictory session.

A report[18] on this Parishad says an appeal was made during the sessions to plan common textbooks for schools in Kochi, Travancore and Malabar; the governments in all three places were requested to compile a dictionary with the cooperation of the Madras University.

P.S. Varier was constantly present at Kailasamandiram on the two days of the Parishad to supervise the arrangements for the invitees and took special interest in the menu for the feasts. He was inordinately pleased that he could be of help to the stars of the literary world. Surely, he thought, it was not given to everyone to have that kind of happiness. The diary entry for 29 December mentions his having a long conversation that afternoon with Ulloor Parameswara Iyer. It gave Varier special pleasure to know that Muslim, Christian and Hindu scholars were all guests under the same roof, that there was no difference between them of class or caste, that they ate and laughed and spoke together like one family.

Varier arranged a special feast for the invitees on the final day. He took care that the needs of each guest were satisfied in every aspect. The vote of thanks spoken that evening acknowledged Varier's hospitality with extravagant praise: the

[18]Chummar, T.M.: *Bhashagadya Sahitya Charithram* (History of Malayalam Prose), Sahitya Pravarthaka Sahakarana Sangham Ltd., National Bookstall, Kottayam, 1955, pp.513-14.

speaker commented that the host had provided each invitee with the particular oil he needed for his bath and the vaka powder or soap to wash it off with such solicitous care that they had all been tempted to wonder whether every guest would also be led to a special bathing tank of his own, with the water in it heated to the precise temperature his body needed![19]

So Kailasamandiram was most unexpectedly inaugurated before it was quite ready. Now P.S. Varier had to turn his attention to the formal inauguration, to the festive celebrations that were going to mark its transformation into a family home.

---

[19] F.: 'Kottakkal', *Souvenir of Vaidyaratnam P.S. Varier's Centenary Celebration*, 1969.

15

The Sixtieth Birthday

Since P.S. Varier's birth star, Ashwini, occurred twice in the
same month in the year 1929, he actually had two sixtieth
birthdays to celebrate. He let the first one go by without any
fanfare, choosing to set it apart for the rituals he wished to
perform. He made offerings in the temples in Kottakkal on
this day. There were two special offerings of money: one to
the Venkitta Thevar temple next to the variam, the temple
where his family had first been given a kazhagam, for renovating
its gopuram and laying copper plates over it; the second
towards repairs which were urgently necessary for the oldest
mosque in Kottakkal, the Palappra mosque. A sloka composed
by Varier was carved on the wall of the Venkitta Thevar
temple on this occasion:

> *Muniyogya samarambha sankaro deva kinkara*
> *Navina makaro dethal mahadevasya mantapam*

(Sankara, the servant of God, has renovated this mantapam of
Mahadeva, a task that only sages are worthy of doing.)

Varier also set aside the money he wanted to send as offerings to the Nelluvaya Dhanvanthari temple, where he had spent his last year of study, and to the old family temple in Nanmanda, the original home of the Panniyampally Variers.

He went to the southern variam to ask his Cheriyamma, Kutty Varasyar, who was now eighty-six, for her blessing and had lunch there. Since his mother's death, it was this beloved Cheriyamma who had served him lunch on every birthday and both were overcome by emotion, aware that this was a particularly significant occasion.

It was a hundred and thirty years since Varier's family had first come to Kottakkal. It was Manorama Thambatti of the eastern kovilakam who had first brought them there. In acknowledgement of this, Varier organized a grand feast for everyone at the kovilakam, including all their employees and dependents.

On 6 April 1929, Varier conducted the grihapravesham ceremony in Kailasamandiram. At the auspicious hour of three-thirty at dawn that day, he, all the members of the family and all the employees in the various establishments gathered at the house and chanted a prayer together. Varier had composed this verse himself and it appears on the right hand corner of the entry in his diary for 5 April 1929:

Kailasagehamithilullu pinakkamenna-
Maleshidhathakhila saukhamanaykkuvanum
Ma leshamullathinu pushtiyinakkuvanum
Shaileshanandini! sadapi thunaykkanam nee

(Parvathi, Daughter of the Mountains, bless and protect me always, so that no sorrows touch this house, so that I have every kind of happiness, so that the auspicious qualities of this house grow stronger.)

The verse showing the kalidinasamkhya of Kailasamandiram, which incorporates the year in which it was built, is inscribed at the entrance to the house. Once again, it was Varier who

composed it and the verse can be seen in the diary entry for
6 April 1929:

Sree varaha viharakhye
Sreevara sangadaayini
Kaliheene nave harmye
Sankarapravishalsukham

(Sankara enters with happiness this new house, the home of
the wild boar, ['the home of the wild boar' refers to Varier's
family name, Panniyinpally; 'panni' is a wild boar, 'pally' is
house or home] which has been blessed by everything auspicious
and which nothing evil or inauspicious can touch.)

The 'kalidinasamkhya' means that the date when the house
was built can be calculated backward from the present from
the arrangement of the letters. Classical scholars of the time
took delight in composing verses incorporating this calculation.
Each letter of the Malayalam alphabet corresponds to a numeral
and the letters to be decoded in this verse are those of the
second line, 'sreevarasangadayini.' The calculation is made as
follows: to the present year, the year 1176 of the Malayalam
era, add the numerals that correspond to the letters in
'taralangam', that is ta, ra, la, ga, read backward, which make
3926. This is now multiplied by the figures corresponding to
'kalohalabham', which brings us to the figure 22,36,25,762.
This figure has to be divided by 120 and becomes 18,63,548.
The numerals corresponding to 'sreevarasangadayini', that is,
18,37,242, have to be subtracted from this. The answer is
26,306, which is the number of days in the required date.
Divided by 365, this gives 72.26. The year 1176 minus 72 years
brings us to the figure 1104 (1929 of the Christian era), the year
in which Kailasamandiram was built.

There was a feast for lunch in Kailasamandiram on the day
the family first entered the house. The women moved in on 8
April and Varier on 13 April.

Varier speaks of his new cot in the diary entry on 9 April, no doubt the brass cot he had sent from Spencer's, Madras:

9 April 1929

In the afternoon, I lay down for two and a half hours on the new cot. It feels very comfortable.

The tenth of April, the second time the star Ashwini occurred that month, was the official date marking P.S. Varier's sixtieth birthday. But the celebrations began a week before the actual day.

4 April 1929

... Gave all the workers lunch. Cooked seven sacks of rice for them.

Tea parties were organized over the week, even before the birthday, each evening being allotted to schoolchildren and teachers from different schools in the village. These included the Kottakkal High School, the Board Hindu Higher Elementary School and the Girls' School on the first day and the Board Mapilla Higher Elementary School on the second day.

On 10 April, P.S. Varier received felicitations and gifts from the many guests who came to wish him, including various members of the extended family who had come from distant villages. By evening, Kailasamandiram came alive with glittering electric lights charged by a dynamo that Varier had specially ordered for the occasion. Crowds flocked to the yard of the house to see this novel and wonderful sight.

More than six hundred Variers had come from different places and there were many women among them. After a splendid feast, Varier gave the prescribed dakshinas to the Brahmins and priests, a dakshina of a silver rupee to all the Variers and a sovereign each to those among them who had turned ninety. Apart from the feast for the invitees, all the people in the village and neighbouring areas were served a feast at which everyone ate together with no distinction of caste and creed. Two hundred paras (a para holds approximately 12 kilograms) of rice were cooked on the ocassion.

The meeting in the evening started at four o'clock. Many local dignitaries and the representatives of various communities gathered to attend it. Letters had been received from hundreds of well-wishers.

The Varier Samajam presented P.S. Varier with a beautiful statue of Dhanvanthari carved in sandalwood. Of the many speeches that were made, the *Shashti Varshika Charithram*, the volume that Varier's students prepared for the occasion, cites the one delivered by T.S. Varier, the representative of the Variers of the Irinjalakuda and Perumanam villages as particularly apt. The speaker points out that P.S. Varier's successes are especially commendable because he achieved them in the teeth of a multitude of obstacles and urges that all young men learn from the story of his life, which teaches that ordinary men can rise to greatness through unselfish action. Managalapatrams were offered after the speeches were over.

Late in the evening, the Mapillas did the kolkali dance, and a Christian group from Thrissur did a tiger dance. At night, the Parama Shiva Vilasam Natakam Company performed the *Prahlada Charitham*, which Varier had written himself. The students and teachers of vaidyam in Varier's Patasala released the *Shashtivarshika Charithram*, (The History of Sixty Years), an account of his life and achievements until then.

All Varier's employees were given a raise in salary in keeping with their designation. Senior employees like Shinnan Menon, who had been in service for a long time, were presented gold medals.

The *Malayala Manorama* of 10 April wished P.S. Varier continued success in his praiseworthy endeavours, the chief of which they described as a determination to give free treatment to the afflicted, and an effort to obtain for Ayurveda whatever useful and applicable help the modern sciences could give it. The *Mathrubhumi* commented that there were few Malayalis outside the government service or law who had progressed as far as Varier had in life by dint of their intelligence and personal efforts. Further, they added, he had in this way been able to contribute greatly to the general good of Kerala.

The celebrations held for the shashtiabdapoorthi, the sixtieth birthday, highlight the image of a man who had not only reaped success and fame in his chosen field, but had won the respect and affection of peers and employees alike. A man who had become something of a legend in his own lifetime, as much to those who shared his life and had the opportunity to witness his everyday activities as to those who saw and admired him from a distance.

It was the day after his sixtieth birthday that A.C. Achuthan Nair, the actor, chose to leave the drama troupe and go away.

11 April 1929

A.C. went away to Tirur without telling me, succumbing to the persuasion of a man named K. Padmanabaha Menon. Sreedharan saw him and brought him back. I sent for the sub-Inspector and told him what had happened. Anyway, I asked them to see if they could bring Padmanabha Menon here. I called A.C. and advised him.

Achuthan Nair's apprenticeship in Sanskrit began very soon after this.

15 April

Made A.C. read three verses from the Bhagavad Gita. I think he will learn the Sanskrit alphabet quickly.

17 April

A.C. seems eager to study. He has started to read the Nagari script. He does not talk about going away now.

He said all he wanted to do was learn pranayamam and things like that.

Achuthan Nair learnt Sanskrit with P.S. Varier for three years, then went on to study vaidyam at the Patasala.

P.S. Varier himself had begun to nurture a secret dream over the past few years: that, after his sixtieth birthday, he would detach himself from this flurry of activity that had become his daily routine, retreat into a quiet life, spend his time in prayer and meditation. He had no immediate family whose welfare he needed to be anxious about, no close ties that claimed his attention. Around this time, he had a photograph taken of himself clad in the traditional mundu and head-scarf of bark that ascetics wear. But although he found the idea of becoming an ascetic attractive in itself, the corollary it entailed, of detaching himself from the Arya Vaidya Sala and the Patasala, the children of his mind and heart, was certainly not one that enchanted him.

Varier had conscientiously tried to remind himself constantly of his shortcomings and endeavour to mend them; to respond with friendliness even to those who showed anger against him; to extend whatever help he could to everyone, irrespective of their caste and creed. Although he felt he had succeeded in overcoming evil emotions to a great extent, he knew for certain that he would never be able to give up his concern for the Arya Vaidya Sala. Even if he were to go to the peaks of the Himalayas and immerse himself in meditation, he knew that the faintest whisper hinting at the disintegration of the Arya Vaidya Sala was sure to shatter his concentration, bring him back to work for its renewal. How then could he ever hope to become a sanyasi? Worse, in the interests of the Vaidya Sala, he was aware that he would even stoop to anger, to praise, to reprimand, none of which were reactions befitting an ascetic.

Until his sixtieth birthday, he had toyed with these

conflicting ideas and imagined he would find a way to resolve them. The moment had come to take a decision, to choose his path. He realized that he was essentially a karmayogi, committed to the path of action and incapable of deviating from it—that ultimately, the way of the ascetic would never be his. He could not give up the Vaidya Sala, its welfare lay too close to his heart. After all, it was a unique establishment—nothing like it had ever flourished in Malabar before, perhaps not even in south India. It was proving of great use not only to the local people but to many people in very distant places who used its services. It had successfully replaced the old, outmoded, cumbersome methods of having Ayurvedic medicines made at home—indeed, such methods had even been forgotten through long disuse. Vaidyans who were Varier's contemporaries had themselves begun to buy the medicines he made, or started to advise their patients to buy them. Thanks to the increased work the Arya Vaidya Sala now had to do, more avenues of employment had become available to the local people and even to people from neighbouring villages. The Patasala was producing vaidyans who would take the learning they had received there to places outside Kerala. The number of poor people who came to the Charitable Hospital was steadily mounting.

Meanwhile, the expenses for running the Patasala were increasing every year. The money Varier used for these expenses came entirely from the profits the Arya Vaidya Sala made. If he were to abandon the Patasala now, thought P.S. Varier, and if it were to crumble because he had abandoned it, would he not be to blame? True, there were now many responsible people to whom he could hand over the reins of administration. But he had not yet indicated to any of them how the wealth he had amassed by dint of his hard work and single-minded devotion should be used after his time for the good of the causes he had espoused so passionately. Time, events, the comments people around him sometimes made had all convinced him that he had to make it clear that the earnings from the Arya Vaidya Sala had to be kept absolutely separate from the family wealth and used solely for propagating the cause of Ayurveda. Until he was satisfied that none of his establishments would be endangered by his moving away from them, he felt he had to continue carrying out his duties. Asceticism, he realized, was not in his destiny. The verse he wrote in his diary at this time expressed these emotions:

Kailasmandiramithil sukhamaryavaidya
Shalasamedhavidhathil manassu vechum
Lolasmanvitha mukundapadam smaricchum
Leelasamethaminivazhanamulla kalam

(Let me live the rest of my days in happiness in this mansion called Kailasamandiram, attending as I should to the running of the Arya Vaidya Sala, while I meditate joyfully, with no other cares, on the feet of Lord Mukundan who stands beside Lakshmi.)

Meanwhile, Varier had decided to build a small temple adjacent to Kailasamandiram, laid the foundation stone for it in February 1929 and ordered the idol he was going to instal in it from Agra. It was to be a four-armed image fashioned in white marble, each of the arms bearing a conch, a discus, a club and a lotus: Vishnu in the form of Vishvambharan. There was a slight variation: the club was in the right hand and the lotus in the left. When the parcel arrived from Agra, Varier instructed that it should be taken to the anteroom of his bedroom, where he usually did his meditation. He had decided to place it in a glass case and worship it there until the temple was ready. The parcel was brought to Kailasamandiram one evening at the hour of dusk. Quite by coincidence, as the statue was lifted out of its wrappings to be transported upstairs, one of the young girls in the family came to the entrance with a lighted oil lamp in her hand—it is a custom in Kerala to light an oil lamp and bring it to the front of the house at twilight, for all the members of the family to worship the flame. So perfectly was this timed that auspicious evening that it seemed as if the lamp had been brought there intentionally to welcome the statue and light its way up the stairs.

P.S. Varier composed two verses in honour of this deity. The first was:

Shivositvam shaktirasi
Sakshannarayanopyasi
Yadatraishvara chaitanyam
Thalsarvam tvayi vidyate

(Lord, You whose nature is auspicious and full of power, You are Narayanan himself. All things that are filled with prosperity in this world, likewise all things that are filled with radiance—they melt into You)

He is said to have chanted this verse fifty thousand times in order to give it power and radiance. He used to chant this and another verse he composed in praise of Vishvambharan every day:

Visvodaya sthitilaya prabhave, svapada
Visvasinamamritadaya chaturbhujaya
Vishvambharodharanayogya suvigrahaya
Vishvambharaya vibhave vidhivannamostu

Vishvasinama seshanam
Ashvasada dayanidhe
Vishambhara! Hrishikesha!
Sashvatham dehi nah sukham

(You who are the reason for the birth of the world, for its continuance and for the deluge that destroys it—as One who grants salvation to all who stand at your feet, firm in their faith, as One with four hands, and a strong and beautiful body that can rule the world and liberate it, as One who fills all spaces everywhere, as Vishvambharan, ruler of the world, may my obeisances come to you in a manner that befits you.

You who give comfort to all who believe in you, O Merciful One! Vishvambhara! Hrishikesha! Give us eternal happiness.)

From the time it was occupied, Kailasamandiram was a lively mansion and quickly became the centre from which Varier's multiple activities radiated. The Arya Vaidya Sala was just next door and employees, visitors and patients could go to and fro without even having to cross the street. The students of the Patasala gathered in Varier's room upstairs to be taught by him; he took Anatomy classes for them and also taught them about the diseases of the nervous system. The actors of the drama company practised in the compound of Kailasamandiram with the musicians and orchestra accompanying them and Varier often joined them, to teach and advise them, to explain various aspects of theatre, elucidating details they could not understand. Sometimes he asked the members of the troupe to go to his sitting room upstairs. Seated in his easy chair, with all of them gathered around him, he would teach them how to sing a new song he had composed for a play.

The younger boys in the drama troupe were everywhere, playing, quarrelling, running errands, filling the compound of Kailasamandiram with noise and laughter. The sharp, hot odours of medicinal brews simmering in wooden vats over the fires in the Arya Vaidya Sala mingled with mouth-watering scents from the northern wing of Kailasamandiram, as the actors sat down to enjoy yet another meal . . .

In the September of 1929, a few months after the family had occupied it, the first family wedding was conducted in Kailasamandiram—Padmavathy Varasyar, the granddaughter of Lakshmi Varasyar, was married to Thrikkovil Achutha Varier. The wedding took place amidst great festivitiy and rejoicing.

There is an amusing incident associated with the wedding. The drama company had suspended its activities for the season, all the stage settings and props had been dismantled and stored away. A large group of Varier women who had come for the wedding were determined to see a performance. They requested Lakshmi Varasyar to arrange one for them and she, in turn, took what she thought was a simple request to her brother, P.S. Varier. Varier, of course, knew that the drama troupe was not performing for a period; he knew equally well that Shoolapani Varier, his trusted manager, could be depended upon in an emergency. He sent for Shoolapani and told him to arrange for a performance that evening. The unhappy Shoolapani rubbed his hands together nervously, wondering how to explain the situation. Before he could think of what to say and how best to say it, Varier, who was stretched out on his bed, said, '*Valliammal Charithram*, that's the one we'll show them,' turned his face abruptly to the wall and closed his eyes. Poor Shoolapani Varier tried to clear his throat once or twice, loudly, but there was no sign that his master had heard. Knowing there was no way out for him, Shoolapani went down the stairs, rapidly going through all kinds of possibilities in his mind ... At 9.00 that night, the curtain went up on the sets of *Valliammal Charithram* and the Varier women watched in delight as the play unfolded.

Those were the days when the poor who visited the houses of rich jenmis, the landlords, had to take off their shirt, their upper cloth, their slippers at the gate. Ambi Iyer and Varier were standing in the portico of Kailasamandiram one evening when a servant from a neighbouring house came there on an errand. He took off his slippers and was about to creep in, holding them in his hand, when Varier said, 'Look, Ambi, did you see what he's doing?' He turned to the servant. 'What are slippers for, man? To protect your feet, not to hold in your hand! Put them on!' Ambi Iyer laughed and the servant shuffled his feet, baffled and embarrassed. Kailasamandiram was the house of a jenmi, a landlord who broke the rules of his class. In 1905, Varier had already written an article on the necessity of wearing slippers.[19] The last part of it, a passionate appeal for slippers as well as for the cause of women, goes like this:

... I don't think there is any more justice in saying that people should take off their slippers when going into temples or before dignitaries than in saying they should take off the mundu they are wearing. Both are particularly necessary for the protection of the body. But slippers are special and of prime importance. This being the case, it is not at all right for people not to wear slippers all the time, or for some people to try to prohibit them from doing so.

The condition of men in this regard is a little better, that of women is much worse. What we must assume from the present situation is that if Hindu women wear slippers, it might be their fate to be even cast out of the community! Although women do not generally have to walk as much as men, it is certain that slippers are no less necessary for women than for men, for their feet are naturally softer and more vulnerable. We can say with conviction that this is one of the worst curses that women—especially our women—have to bear among many others. Just as in the case of education, slippers are necessary not only for men but for women as well. Therefore we proclaim firmly that all human beings, without prejudice to caste, place or time, should

[19]*Dhanvanthari*, 14 March, 1905.

wear slippers the moment they place their feet on the ground and that people of the older generation, dignitaries and the government, should allow them to do so.

Was there, in this passionate tirade, the echo of a young boy's agony as he tramped barefoot over mile after dusty mile of a rough country road, an enormous sack full of bell-metal vessels that clattered and slid about, balanced precariously on his head?

16

The Temple for Vishvambharan

Once P.S. Varier moved to Kailasamandiram, the students of the Patasala used to gather regularly for classes on the *Ashtangasaareeram* in his sitting room on the first floor. Each student had a duty to perform: placing Varier's chair in position, arranging his books and his writing materials in their places, closing the windows and so on. Aryavaidyan S. Varier, who was one of his students, recalls[20] an incident which brought home to him P.S. Varier's insistence on unvarying routine as discipline. It was S. Varier's responsibility to close the window next to Varier's chair. One day, one of the other students closed the window instead of him, and S. Varier did not pay any great attention to this. After class that morning, P.S. Varier asked: 'What's wrong with your hand, Sankaran?' Puzzled, the boy answered, 'Nothing.' 'I asked because someone else closed the window,' remarked his teacher. Any task, he explained to his young students, had to be carried out by the

---

[20]S. Varier: 'Addeham' (For Him, with Respect), *Souvenir of Vaidyaratnam P.S. Varier's Centenary Celebration*, 1969, p.54.

person who had initially assumed the responsibility for it, no matter how insignificant it seemed, regardless of whether he had been appointed to it or chosen to do it himself, for it played an important role in learning how be disciplined.

S. Varier was a student who had particularly benefited from P.S. Varier's generosity. Repeatedly frustrated in his intense longing to study, forced to content himself to taking occasional lessons with teachers who lived in wealthy houses in the vicinity of his village, never able to learn anything he had started fully, he had listened from the time he was a child to snippets of information about the Patasala at Kottakkal, where students could learn vaidyam free, and longed to go there himself. One of P.S. Varier's students, P.V. Rama Varier, finally took him there, warning him that his application might already be too late for the current year.

S. Varier describes the first time he saw his future teacher.[21]

> The night of 9 June 1927. I stood with the old and new students in front of the Arya Vaidya Chikitsasala by Rama Varier's side. That was the period when he used to spend the night in the room above the Chikitsasala. He came as usual in his car and got down in the porch. Running his eyes quickly over everyone, he walked towards the stairs. He had noticed someone he had not seen there the day before, so he called out while climbing the stairs, 'Who is the new boy with you, Raman?'
>
> I looked at that image for the first time. Fair-skinned and well built. A felt cap on his head. A high forehead, a smiling face. A magnanimous smile. Eyes that brimmed with nobility. Gold-framed glasses. A flannel coat. A pristine white mundu. In his right hand, a

---

[21]Ibid, p.52.

polished black, silver-topped walking stick with a curved handle. Chrome slippers. This was how he looked. Ramettan answered, 'He lives close to my village and is from a poor Varier family. He came with me because he wants to study vaidyam.'

Then he asked me, 'Have you learnt Sanskrit?'

'A little.'

'What have you learnt?'

I mentioned the names of a few poems, of certain cantos in them.

'Will you study well?'

'I will.'

He said to Ramettan, 'Ask Ramunni Menon to enroll him.' By this time he had reached the top of the stairs. That scene, that image, those words remain fresh in my memory.

The boy became one of his most trusted assistants after he qualified, and worked as an Ayurvedic physician in charge of the Palakkad and Kozhikode branches of the Arya Vaidya Sala for many years. He was the chief physician at Kottakkal until he died.

Once he settled down in Kailasamandiram, where he was once again the centre of the family, P.S. Varier was convinced that asceticism was not going to be his chosen way of life and that the first thing he had to do was sort out his financial affairs without too much delay. He also had to think seriously about appointing responsible people to carry on his work. His nephew, Madhavan, had qualified from the Patasala in 1929 and, despite his early ill-health, had done brilliantly. Varier had feared at one time that the boy would not be able to fulfil his duties in life. Besides being weak and sickly, he had been slow to learn and his teachers had been disappointed in him. But

Madhavan's will to overcome his weakness had finally triumphed. On the advice of Meledath Namboodiri, an expert in spells and mantras, Madhavan's father, Talappana Sreedharan Namboodiri, had taught him the bala mantra, which was said to have great power. The boy had chanted it regularly and devotedly for three whole years, isolating himself in a little deserted room directly under the tiled roof of the old variam. His persistence had been rewarded. Varier was confident that he would now be able to take over his responsibilities and administer the establishments he had founded.

The circumstances that turned Varier's thoughts urgently in this direction occurred unexpectedly and were a source of great pain and anxiety to him for a long while. On 14 April 1930, the day of Vishu, the Malayalam New Year, Kutty Varasyar, the Cheriyamma he loved very dearly, talked to him about the debts that her son, P.V. Krishna Varier, had accumulated and asked him to clear them. Varier had already done this once, but thought it would do the family no good if he continued to do so. The diary entry for 14 April 1930 records how deeply the incident shattered him emotionally, since he had not expected his Cheriyamma to confront him as she had done.

14 April 1930

When I went to the variam, Cheriyamma spoke to me about the matter of clearing Kunjukuttan's debts. Although I explained to her that this was not possible and even fell at her feet, she would not agree. I was deeply distressed and felt exhausted, so I went upstairs without even having coffee and lay down, full of sorrow . . . Finally, unable to walk the distance, I sent for the car and then went to the Vaidya Sala.

Varier told his Cheriyamma that the children of the family would eventually starve if he spent money on clearing these debts and assured her that what he desired was the well-being of the whole family, that it could not be risked for the sake of one person. He kept his word and made sure that although P.V. Krishna Varier had to pay the penalty for the debts he incurred, his family did not want for anything and that they always had all they needed to live a comfortable life.

However, the episode led to his feeling so uneasy and vulnerable that he felt even his health had been affected by it. He alludes to this event in the diaries of 1934 and 1935 as one that left him feeling weak over a long period. He knew for certain that the time had come to take decisions about the ownership and administration of his various properties. As a first measure towards this, he drafted a will that was registered on 18 May 1930 and entrusted it to the Registrar's office in Kozhikode for safekeeping. The terms of the will were subsequently altered twice, to make them clearer and more definite and it was the will dated 31 October 1939 that came into operation after his death.

A look at the daily routine described in P.S. Varier's diary at the beginning of the year 1930 offers a picture of the discipline he exercised in his own life:

Permanently settled in the new variam. I get up at 6.00 in the morning, examine my pulse, the specific gravity of my urine and check the temperature outside. I clean my teeth, empty my bowels. Generally, at 7.00, I have coffee and wheat dosais with sugar. Before 7.30 I reach the Vaidya Sala, go through the mail and read the paper. After that, if there is anything particular to write, I finish that. If I have to teach Shareeram, it is at this time that I do so. If I do not have to do either of these, I rest until 9.00. At 9.00 I sign money orders and so on and have coffee, snacks like roasted pappadams and one or two biscuits that do not contain sugar. Then I go down, examine patients and look into the accounts. I go to the hospital if I have to. Otherwise I go straight to the new variam. If there is time, I teach A.C. for a while. At 11.00, I eat cooked wheat with three teaspoons of ghee. Generally, I go easy on red chillies and tamarind. By noon, I close the door and lie down. At 2.00, I dictate replies to the letters received and make Appunni write them down. Usually, this takes an hour and a quarter. Rarely, it takes two and a half hours. I have coffee at 3.30 with a few banana chips or a banana. I then check the mail and read the paper. After 4.00, I examine patients who have come from outside if there are any. I walk around the house for at least a quarter of an hour. At 6.00 in the evening, I have an oil bath. The water is boiled and I have a bath in the bathroom. In cold weather, I use marichaadi oil for the head and manjishtadi oil in hot weather. If I have rheumatic pains, I use balaguluchyadi oil for one or two days and nimbadi thailam if I have dandruff. On the body I generally use dineshavalyaadi and sometimes vathamardanam oil. I use soap to remove the oil and vellila thali for the head. On the first of every Malayalam month, I have a dip in the variam tank and worship in all the temples. Similarly, I have a dip in the tank on shraddham days, on my birthday and on festival days like Thiruvonam. All these baths in the tank are in the mornings and the baths in hot water in the evenings. Every other day, I rub oil over my entire body. On other days, only 'shira shravana paadeshu' (that is, on my head, my ears and my feet). At 6.45 I have coffee and fried pappadams. After that, I say my prayers for fifteen to twenty minutes. Then I read a chapter of the Bhagavatham. Usually, I read a lot of the Gita. It is the prayers that I am very regular about. After 8.30, I have cooked wheat like at 11.00 in the morning, but no ghee. I go upstairs at 9.00. Most days, I teach A.C. for a while. I go to bed at 10.30. On days when I do not teach him, I go to sleep at 9.30. Most days, A.C. sleeps upstairs so that he can be of assistance to me. If he is away, I do not allow anyone else to sleep upstairs. On the first of every month I go to Calicut. On those days, before I go to bed at night, I drink milk. But I do not drink it every day since it increases the formation of phlegm. I take very little sugar, except in the morning, when I take some with wheat dosais—altogether, every day, I take sugar that weighs about a rupee and a quarter (the weight of a rupee coin is about 10 grams). I have about four motions a day usually and pass urine four or five times a day. In summer, I drink tea instead of coffee in the evening. If I feel weak, I take small amounts of dashamoolarishtam.

In 1930, there was a students' demonstration in the Patasala. One of the students came to class wearing a Gandhi cap and was asked to leave. The next day, all the students wore Gandhi caps to class, then staged a demonstration that made its way to the yard of Kailasamandiram. There was no violence, however, and the trouble subsided quickly.

In 1931, a very important vistor came to see P.S. Varier in Kailasamandiram—his old mentor and friend, Dr Verghese. It was an unforgettable occasion for Varier. He presented the doctor with a beautiful cross, fashioned in gold and studded with gems. The event is recorded in his diary:

18 January 1931

Dr Verghese and Madhavan came. We had lunch together, a feast. Had sweet milk payasam made with rice. Presented Dr Verghese with a gold cross.

It was an equally memorable visit for the doctor, an opportunity for him to see for himself how well his student had done, how far he had progressed. A photograph of Dr Verghese now occupies a prominent position on the wall of the sitting room in Kailasamandiram. Over the course of the years, neither family has forgotten the old bond: as recently as two years ago, in 1999, a grandson of the doctor, now settled in England, visited Kerala, remembered the story of his grandfather's disciple and came to Kailasamandiram, with a host of relatives in two cars, to pay a visit to the family.

By this time the Arya Vaidya Sala had become so well known that P.S. Varier kept receiving requests to open branches elsewhere. Although he had thought it was a good thing to open a branch in Kozhikode, since it was the principal town in Malabar, he was not really keen to extend this service further. But many of his patients in Tamil Nadu and his friends in the Palakkad area kept telling him that they would find it a boon to have an Arya Vaidya Sala somewhere in their vicinity. Around this time, Varier happened to hear that the Amity Hall and the power house building in Vadakkanthara in Palakkad were being sold by auction in Court. On 3 January 1932, P.S. Varier bought these buildings in his own name for Rs 10,520. Spending almost as much again, he had the place renovated, added new buildings and opened a branch of the Arya Vaidya Sala on 28 April 1932. P.S. Varier's nephew, Madhava Varier, was appointed to be in charge of this branch. The physician S. Varier notes in his diary that, rather surprisingly, P.S. Varier did not attend the inaugural function. But he began to make fortnightly visits to both branches, at Kozhikode and Palakkad, to see patients there.

The temple for the idol of Vishvambharan was by now ready on the southern side of Kailasamandiram. The idol was brought down from Varier's bedroom and installed in the temple on 1 April 1932. The little temple, perfectly proportioned and set like a jewel in the southern courtyard, was very different from other Kerala temples from the day of its installation, for it was open to all castes. It would be another five years before the Maharaja of Travancore would pass the Temple Entry Act in 1937 and declare the temples in the Travancore district open to all castes and still another ten years from then before the Maharaja of Cochin and the Samoothiri of Kozhikode would follow suit. In addition, men and women in Kottakkal could enter the Vishvambhara temple fully dressed at a period when the dress regulations were very strict in many temples in Kerala. Men could not wear shirts or any other article of clothing that covered their torso within a temple; in some temples, particularly those belonging to the kovilakams, women could not enter wearing blouses. The absence of such restrictions in the Vishvambhara temple drew the attention of the public and the *Mathrubhumi* of 8 April 1932 published the following note:

A NEW TEMPLE WHERE THE INFERIOR CASTES
CAN ENTER
(A Correspondent)

Kottakkal, 6 April: Last Saturday, Sriman P.S. Varier ceremonially installed Lord Dhanvanthari in the temple he has built in his residence, 'Kailasamandiram'. The temple is special in that inferior castes are allowed entry to worship in it. Moreover, it is not forbidden to go to worship fully dressed. The rule that women cannot enter to worship wearing their blouses is still strictly observed in the temples inside the kovilakams. While congratulating Sriman P.S.Varier on his liberal outlook and vision, we respectfully invite the educated and modern inmates of the kovilakams to expedite amendments compatible with our times.

(8.4.1932)

P.S. Varier himself wore a shirt when he went to the Vishvambhara temple. In any case, he showed scant respect for rules of ritual purity which seemed decadent or meaningless to him. One of his grandnephews, Appu, who used to live in the southern variam, used to wait eagerly for him every evening. Varier would go for a walk past the house and, on his way back, he would come in and sit for a while, talking to the child's grandmother, Varier's Cheriyamma. One day, Appu went up to them and his granduncle lifted him onto his lap. Since Varier had been out walking (and with companions whose class and caste might be questionable), Appu's mother and grandmother scolded the child: they would have to give him a bath in the tank now, so late in the evening, for having touched his grand-uncle. Varier smiled and asked them gently whether it was really necessary to submit a four-year-old child to such rigorous rules of ritual purity. His grandmother gave in and waived a bath, but insisted that the shirt the child wore be washed at once. Next evening, when Varier came, he gave Appu a packet and said, 'Wear this, then you won't have to have a bath when you touch me.' The packet contained a silk shirt—silk could not be made impure, according to the rules! Appu Varier affectionately recalls how he wore the silk shirt every evening after that and played with his grand-uncle, sitting on his lap whenever he wanted to.

In 1932, the government instituted the Central Board of Indian Medicine and P.S. Varier was nominated a member. Some years later, when members came to be chosen by election, he offered himself as a candidate and was elected. He was also made an Examiner for the School of Indian Medicine in Madras.

In 1933, in recognition of his remarkable services to the cause of Ayurveda, a great honour was conferred on P.S. Varier—he was awarded the title of 'Vaidyaratnam'. Lord Willingdon, Viceroy and Governor General of India, signed the citation.

‌‍‍‌‍‌‌‍‌

The Venkitta Thevar temple used to give an annual feast to all the Variers, the Pisharotys and other communities who lived around the temple. For some reason, they stopped doing so in 1934. P.S. Varier had already been thinking of having an annual celebration in his own Vishvambhara temple, an event that everyone in Kottakkal and its vicinity would be able to appreciate and enjoy. He decided to institute an annual temple festival that would last seven days, the final ceremonies coinciding with his birthday. The colourful Vishvambhara temple festival that is now an important event in Kerala was first celebrated in 1934. From the beginning, it was conducted on an elaborate scale: there were five to seven caparisoned elephants for the sreebali processions that took place morning and evening, and sixty to seventy drummers participated in the melam that accompanied the processions, the intricate rhythm patterns their drums wove echoing vibrantly through the air. Expert nadaswaram players participated as well. Performances of the temple arts like Ottan Thullal and Chakyar Koothu started in the afternoon on the days of the festival and went on until the evening pujas and processions began. There were spectacular fireworks after that followed by performances of Kathakali that continued throughout the night.

To the great delight of the children in Kailasamandiram, Varier bought a baby elephant around this time and called it Balan. Its gradually increasing height is often noted in the diaries:

28 January 1940
Baby elephant—height 77", back 81". On 10 March 1939, height 75".

13 January 1942
Baby elephant—height 83.5". On 30 January 1941, height 80".

4 January 1944
Baby elephant—height 89". On 5 January 1943, height 86".

Varier was very fond of Balan and the elephant, treated by everyone with great affection, knew and loved everyone in Kailasamandiram in return. He was sold after Varier's death in 1944 and taken away from Kottakkal. It is said that he was brought back once, for the temple festival. A few miles from Kottakkal, Balan realized where he was going, walked rapidly away from his mahout and arrived by himself in the courtyard of the Vishvambhara temple! Excited to be back, he walked around Kailasamandiram, stopping at the back door, where he remembered Kunji Varasyar holding out a bunch of bananas to him . . .

Much earlier, Keshavan, the famous elephant from the Guruvayoor temple, was once brought to Kottakkal for the festival there. It ran amuk one morning and Shoolapani Varier, terrified, rushed up the stairs in Kailasamandiram to tell P.S.Varier what had happened. He found Varier standing at the window enjoying the spectacle of Keshavan running all over the courtyard. 'Why are you so worried?' he asked the incoherent Shoolapani, 'Keshavan's mahout is there, he'll look after him.'

The little village of Kottakkal was by now known all over India. In Kottakkal itself, P.S. Varier, his house, his car, his friends, his principal employees were all enveloped in an aura of charm and magic that they wore with light-hearted pride. Varier's evening walks with his companions, his car rides, became part of the life of Kottakkal. As did the style of dress he adopted when he went out: a felt cap or a cap-like turban on his head, a coat with a gold-bordered angavastram draped over it, trousers and shoes. His regular food habits were frugal and planned to be healthy. But he loved Nice biscuits (that were lightly sprinkled with sugar), probably ordered from Madras. He records eating these in his diaries from time to time, as he also records the days on which he ate ice cream, obviously a delicacy he enjoyed.

After moving to Kailasamandiram, Varier began to give all his relatives and employees, including the employees of the Kottakkal post office, the Registrar's office, the railway station and the police station new clothes every year for Onam, the annual harvest festival that is celebrated throughout Kerala in August-September, a tradition that still continues.

Students who had learnt vaidyam from him began to come every year on the last day of Navarathri, Vijayadashami day, for the Vidyarambham ceremony. It is considered auspicious for students to learn from their guru on that day. Everyone assembled in Varier's sitting room upstairs in Kailasamandiram. Varier would sit with his legs crossed, on a low wooden stool on the ground, a stack of palm-leaf manuscripts beside him, many of which were from the *Ashtangahridayam*. His students, including senior vaidyans who had studied under him, would come one by one in order of seniority and be given a manuscript. He would then read out certain verses and they would repeat them. S. Varier mentions in his diaries that P.S. Varier observed this ceremony even on an occasion when he was not well, on Vijayadashami day in 1939, when, unable to sit on the ground, he conducted it from an easy chair.

Everyone who worked with Varier learnt to respect his demands for perfection and the subtle ways in which he imposed them. Shoolapani Varier, the manager of the drama troupe, who had to deal with him many times every day in the course of his multifarious duties, realized very early that he could not afford to be forgetful or slipshod. One evening, in the days before Shoolapani Varier had fully understood what was expected of him, he came up to P.S. Varier's room in Kailasamandiram and was asked what play the drama troupe was performing that night. Shoolapani rushed down to find out, since he had not checked what the actors had been

rehearsing and ran back up the stairs to tell P.S. Varier what
the play was. Varier nodded his head. 'And who is doing the
lead role?' he asked, with studied casualness. Shoolapani pelted
down the stairs again, why had he not thought of finding out?
He came back, gasping. P.S. Varier had not moved from his
chair. 'What about the two women—who is doing their roles?'
From that day onwards, Shoolapani Varier never went up to
discuss the plays without first making sure he knew all the
details of the production! Eventually, Varier found Shoolapani
Varier so dependable that he gave him many responsibilities
besides the drama troupe—like the management of the accounts
for the temple and its annual festival and for all the meals
served in Kailsamandiram to the employees and guests.

Shoolapani Varier's diaries, which he started to write in
1929 and continued until the sixties, testify to the meticulous
manner in which he kept accounts and to the sincerity with
which he carried out his duties. They record the most minute
details of expenditure, including trifling sums he spent on his
laundry and other personal needs. They are proof of the time
he spent looking after the concerns of the drama troupe, from
arranging their food and accommodation to supervising the
arrangements in the hall, helping to draft and print the notices
and—not least of all—mediating in the petty quarrels and
arguments that constantly erupted among the members of the
organization. Most nights, the diaries record his having gone to
bed at one or two in the early hours of the morning, no doubt
after the evening's performance. He complains often of a
headche, of not feeling well, most of all, of being distressed or
worried about something that was not going right. Inclined to
be tense and vulnerable, he was obviously easily upset, especially
because he tried to solve most of the problems that came his
way himself, not wanting to disturb P.S. Varier. It was said
that he used to buy the actors a drink now and then, to keep
them in good humour and because he felt they needed it, but

that he never entered the amounts he spent this way in the accounts.

As he grew older, Varier became increasingly concerned with his health and wrote very detailed accounts of it in his diaries. The first section in each diary, before the entry for 1 January began, usually described his physical condition during the year that had just passed. The diary of 1935 has a particularly long description of his state of health from 1927 to 1935 and reveals his anxiety about the sugar detected in his urine.

> 1925 and the beginning of 1926. Worked very hard on the *Ashtangashareeram*. Sat in the same spot and worked 10 to 12 hours . . .

> 1926 August. Had urine examined by Dr Venkatachala Iyer. Specific gravity 1024°. A little sugar detected.

> 1927 September. Had urine tested in the Kozhikode hospital. Specific gravity 1027°. The result they wrote was: Reaction acid. Albumin nil. Sugar present, 9.825 grs. per oz. From that evening, began to cut down on red chillies and tamarind in food.

> From 25 September, made it a rule to take wheat for one meal a day.

> 1927 October. Began to take wheat twice a day. From that time, the specific gravity of urine began to go down rapidly. For two days, it was only 1012.

The preoccupation with the figures indicating the specific gravity of his urine became a regular feature of the diaries. The recordings of the most minute variations in the figures and the consequent changes Varier immediately made in his diet are proof of the attention he unfailingly paid to his health. He knew that the enormity of the duties he had taken upon himself as his establishments expanded could be a drain on his health—and he was not getting any younger.

In the diary entry for 29 September 1935, he composed two eloquent verses, one in Malayalam and the other in Sanskrit, in which he expressed his distress at having had to shoulder the burden of being the serniormost male member of the family, the karanavan:

Karanavan jnanennoru
Dharanakondanu chodikkunnathenkil
Maranaminimelvenda
Karanammozhiyunnu jnanitha

(If you ask me because I am the seniormost male member, the karanavan of the family—what a nuisance! Don't ask any more, I am giving up my position now.)

Yathashakthi svakrithyani nissahayo vinirvahal
Kathanjithiha jeevami sarvam vishvambhare arpayan
Tasyamenaparadhasya manahkshobhayithum muhu
Yatateyasyasyegathi kavasyannarakarithe

(Even though I have no one to help me, I manage somehow. I lay everything at Vishvambharan's feet and perform all my duties to the best of my strength. Whoever tries to provoke the anger of a faultless person like this will be destined to endure hell).

He had already written a will by this time and was obviously anxious to give up responsibilities which weighed heavily on him.

In 1936, P.S. Varier's beloved Cheriyamma, Kutty Varasyar, died, at the age of ninety-three. She had taken his mother's place for many years and her death was a great blow to him.

Although Varier's routine remained regular and he adhered scrupulously to his frugal food habits, his evening walks and his oil baths, a fatigue took possession of him by 1937. He refused to give in to it, however, and kept thinking of ways to

overcome it. It was at this time that he came across a news item
in the papers: that Pandit Madan Mohan Malaviya had begun
to take the kaya kalpa treatment prescribed in Ayurveda for
rejuvenation, but that he had not been able to complete it.
P.S. Varier's thoughts turned immediately in this direction.
The regimen the treatment required was extremely severe.
Because of this, and because of the complicated procedures that
were part of this rasayana form of treatment, it was very seldom
practised. But Varier thought of the difficulties it presented as
a challenge. He became increasingly convinced that this
treatment would definitely lessen the fatigue that was plaguing
him and give him a new lease of health and physical strength.

He therefore started the treatment on 23 January 1938. He
chose the 'Brahmarasayanam', which had been prescribed by
the sages as efficacious for radiant health and longevity. He had
designed the treatment room in his suite in Kailasamandiram
specifically for long-term types of treatment like this and it was
therefore done there.

Varier observed almost all the rules of the diet and regimen
prescribed for the treatment, but found it impossible to give up
certain activities that were actually forbidden—like drafting
replies to a few important letters from patients, examining a
patient or two who, he felt, really required advice and treatment
urgently and walking for a short while around the Vishvambhara
temple in the evenings. He wrote regularly in his diary as well.

The chosen rasayanam is the only intake the patient
following this treatment is allowed to have. Starting with small
quantities, it is increased according to the demands of the
patient's digestive system. Only after the rasayanam that is
taken early morning is digested can the patient drink even
boiled, cooled water. P.S. Varier followed this strict regime for
twenty-one days, then observed a period of rest that lasted
forty days. At the end of the two months, he felt that his
mental and physical capacities had improved remarkably and

that his mind was extraordinarily at peace. His face is said to have acquired a radiance that touched all those around him.

In September 1938, Jaya Prakash Narayan came to Kottakkal for treatment, advised to do so by Gandhiji. Long periods in jail, when he was confined in a cell with a cement floor, had resulted in the arthritic pains which had brought Narayan to Kottakkal. N.V. Krishnankutty Warrier, the Ayurvedic scholar, was then a young boy. He and a group of other young boys decided to form a guard of honour at the crossroads leading to Kottakkal and give J.P. Narayan a reception.[22]

Krishnankutty Warrier discovered that Narayan had not decided on a place to stay and suggested that he and his wife, who had come with him, stay on the ground floor of an old building where he lived with his family, since it was lying vacant. Young Krishnankutty was then in the fifth form in school. He attended on all Narayan's needs and enjoyed the excitement in the house when many Congress leaders visited Narayan.

On 30 October 1939, P.S. Varier, now seventy years old, recorded an important happening in his diary:

30 October 1939

Signed at dusk, at 7.15, on the new will.

This was the will that became effective after his death.

In the introductory pages in the diary for 1940, Varier again summarizes recent happenings:

---

[22]From a conversation with Sri N.V. Krishnankutty Warrier at the Arya Vaidya Sala, Kottakkal in January 2001.

1939 was a year in which many important things happened. From 1926, there was a little sugar—2.75 per cent in the urine. But there were no other ailments to speak of. By the end of 1938, I became very weak. In January, I could not walk the usual 12 miles—I could hardly manage 3 miles. Weighed only 146 lbs.

He goes on to speak of how he began to take Brahmarasayanam and how this made him feel very much better. At the beginning of 1940, Varier notes:

1 January 1940

The ache and weakness in my right hand has not fully disappeared. Although the general weakness is much less, my hand aches if I use a walking stick, so I am not able to walk as much as usual.

Age was certainly beginning to tell on Varier's physical condition. Although he wisely decided to curtail his activities, the tone of the diary entries betrays a regret in having been obliged to do so.

17

A Renaissance Personality

What was it that made P.S. Varier so radically different from the vaidyans of his time? Perhaps the answer is that his vision was not confined to the period he lived in, it spanned all time. A boundless curiosity that propelled him into learning whatever he could about everything going on in the world and a determination to make all that he learnt an integral part of his own world gave his vision a range and scope that were unique.

One of the most important facets of Varier's personality was his considered acceptance of the tradition he was born into. In a series of articles called 'Western and Eastern Medicine' he dealt at length with the origin of Ayurveda. He was certain that the gods had gifted Ayurveda to human beings:

> What we call Ayurveda is the sum of all the collected knowledge we need about longevity. This knowledge is true, eternal and permanent. It is surmised that the creator of the universe and the creator of this Ayurveda are the same. What we understand from the shastrams, our scriptures, is that at the same moment that God

decided to create human beings, he was anxious about
the dangers that might befall them and created Ayurveda
as a remedy for these dangers.[23]

Varier was equally certain that in the course of time, because
of the carelessness and indifference of the people who practised
it, a number of shortcomings had come to be associated with
this divine gift. These shortcomings had not been taken note
of or rectified because an attitude of complacency had crept
into the system. One of the aspects of western medicine that
Varier admired and appreciated deeply was the climate of
questioning which nourished it and contributed richly to its
constant growth and improvement. Varier believed that
Ayurveda could not evolve unless it learned to question its
tenets and practices in a similar manner.

It could be said that there were, at the time when Varier
began to learn vaidyam and practise it, three kinds of indigenous
physicians: those who were rigidly and uncompromisingly
orthodox and for whom western medicine did not exist at all,
those who were influenced by western medicine, and those
who condemned western medicine completely. P.S. Varier did
not fit into any of these categories. He thought of Ayurveda as
a perfect health care system that had been explicitly devised to
benefit the Indian physique. He also felt that this system had
been gradually disintegrating because of the indifference of its
practitioners and that it could be meaningfully revived by
adopting methods and principles from western medicine that
would revitalize it. A.C. Achuthan Nair speaks of how P.S.
Varier once told him that he was willing to adopt any procedures
in western medicine that would give a patient relief.

The first step he took in this direction, completely on his
own initiative, by opening a centre that processed and sold

---

[23]Varier P.S.: 'Western and Eastern Medicine', *Dhanvanthari*, 1914.

indigenous medicines, was of crucial importance to his cause. Most people had realized that processing medicines at home was a lengthy, cumbersome and expensive affair. To be able to buy them ready-made, to be assured that they had been processed under expert supervision and that their quality was excellent: these were advantages that no one, rich or poor, could ignore for long. Varier had become aware of this as soon as he began to practise vaidyam and had wasted no time at all in trying to find ways and means to carry out his aim. He had therefore displayed an extraordinarily sharp insight into the situation he found himself in when he came back to settle down in Kottakkal. He had set aside his second ambition, to found an institution that would offer an organized system to study vaidyam, for the moment. He knew it was a project that would take time to consolidate—besides, it would not benefit such a large section of people immediately as the establishment of a vaidya sala undoubtedly would.

From its inception, the Arya Vaidya Sala organized a mail order system that was novel and wide-reaching. The special attention Varier paid to this aspect of the Vaidya Sala is evident in the regularity with which he maintained it, personally attending to letters and replies, until his death. His diaries carry every day, without exception, the sentence, 'Read letters, drafted replies, signed V.P. forms.' As he grew older and began to delegate responsibilities to trusted assistants, he mentions that it was Madhavan (his nephew and the first managing trustee) who signed the forms. The fourth edition, revised and enlarged, of the *Chikitsasamgraham*, published in 1933, includes a long list of requirements for letters sent by patients. Varier explains that the details given by patients in their letters are often insufficient and asks for specific information that will help diagnosis and treatment. Besides basic facts like age, sex and the symptoms and history of illness, Varier asks for a description of the patient's daily routine, the state of his appetite, an account of his temperament, his idiosyncrasies, the kind of environment he lives in, his financial status, whether he has a physician within reach; if the patient is a woman, he aks for details of their menstrual cycles, pregnancies and childbirths. He then invites patients to mention other details that might seem relevant to their particular ailment. The letters could therefore be very lengthy. Varier trained his staff to abridge them, and present the salient facts to him during the sessions he spent going through this correspondence. Until his death in 1944, he attended to the replies himself. This practice of treatment by correspondence still continues and the Arya Vaidya Sala receives letters from and sends replies to patients all over the world.

The various stages of planning that engaged Varier while organizing the Patasala can be easily followed: the proceedings of the Arya Vaidya Samajam and various articles in the *Dhanvanthari* describe them clearly. The Arya Vaidya Sala, however, was started so early in Varier's career and adopted what must have certainly been a well-planned line of action so quickly and smoothly, targeting large numbers of buyers inside and outside Kerala, that it is only possible to guess at the kind of obstacles Varier must have faced and surmounted as a very young man in the course of its establishment.

As time went on, the ability Varier possessed to set in motion whole chains of activities that were complete in themselves and intricately connected to one another as well, developed to an amazing degree and grew increasingly sophisticated. The Parama Shiva Vilasam Nataka Company, which was started to provide temporarily unemployed workers of the Vaidya Sala a livelihood expanded into a full-fledged theatre company that played to audiences throughout Kerala. Varier trained his actors with such care and paid such close attention to details like props, settings and music that the troupe could soon hold its own against much older, established

Tamil theatre companies. The *Dhanvanthari* magazine became a forum for lively and critical debate on controversial issues that involved the entire medical profession. Kailasamandiram, from the time it was occupied, became a centre for cultural activities that drew participants from within and outside Kerala. The drama troupe and the magazine, besides fulfilling their main functions, also acted as publicity agents for the Arya Vaidya Sala. If all these institutions, all these activities, had capable managers at their helm, it is also true that Varier never relaxed his vigilance over any of them. He had obviously inherited his mother's phenomenal memory and efficiency: nothing and no one in the vast domain he supervised in Kottakkal escaped his attention.

Any movement that he initiated assumed social, intellectual and cultural dimensions that rapidly went beyond the context they were conceived in, making each of them what the historian K.N. Panikkar calls 'part of a multi-pronged cultural endeavour' that embraced a distinctively Kerala culture. In this sense, Varier can best be described as a true Renaissance figure. Constantly forging ahead of his contemporaries, he was equally fascinated by the arts and the sciences. Deeply rooted in tradition, trained in classical Sanskrit, dedicated as a student to the ancient gurukulam method of learning, he was always intensely aware of all the novel trends in literature, the arts and medicine. Curious by nature, restless for knowledge, he was daring in his ambitions, avid for perfection. He believed and tried to demonstrate that what was traditional in India could be revitalized, recharged by western thoughts and ideas that could be adapted to the demands of Ayurveda. Side by side, he wanted everyone to understand and appreciate the time-honoured principles and practices in Ayurveda and the classical arts and literatures of India.

Varier could turn his gift for writing to a variety of subjects: tracts on diseases he had seen and worked with, like cholera and the plague; instructions on how to manage

pregnancy and childbirth, how to arrange a room for an
invalid; textbooks in Malayalam and in Sanskrit that would
help students of vaidyam; essays and articles that propagated
the cause of Ayurveda. The *Brihadshareeram* is decribed as
'scientific, precise, syncretic and heavily illustrated' by Dominik
Wujastyk,[24] who goes on to say that the *Brihadshareeram* and
Gananath Sen's *Prathyakshashareeram* (which P.S. Varier used
in the Patasala) are 'earnest and philosophically informed and
the product of real learning,' especially when compared to later
works by other authors that show a lack of interest in
observation and comparative anatomy. Varier could handle
other kinds of writing with equal ease: he composed plays and
songs in Malayalam, translated prose and verse from Sanskrit.
He was the phenomenon known as a nimishakavi: he could
toss off a verse to suit any situation in a minute. His long poem
on Vishnu, the *Bhagavad Keshadipadam*, an eloquent physical
description of the deity from head to foot, published in the
Mathrubhumi weekly in 1940, is sung now in the Vishvambhara
temple.

Varier was far ahead of his time in his attitude towards
caste and religion. At a time when the caste system was
extremely rigid and severe in Kerala and the rules of ritual
purity blindly enforced, people of all castes were welcome in
Kailasamandiram and the Vishvambhara temple was open to
anyone who wished to worship. This was much before the
Temple Entry Act allowed people of all castes into the Kerala
temples. At the time of the Mapilla revolt in 1921, the Arya
Vaidya Sala became home to Hindus and Muslims alike. Over
the arched gateway of Kailasamandiram, Hindu, Muslim and
Christian symbols are drawn over a verse that says:

---

[24]Wujastyk, Dominik: 'Interpreting the Image of the Human Body in
Pre-Modern India' in *Les Representations du Corps dans le Monde
Hindou*, Paris, CNRS editions, forthcoming.

Dharmojayathi nadharma
Satyam jayathi nanritham
Kshama jayathi nakrodho
Vishnur jayathi napara

(Only dharma can triumph, adharma cannot; only truth can triumph, untruth cannot; only patience can triumph, anger cannot; only Vishnu can triumph, no one else can.)

Varier had an easy, affectionate, deeply personal relationship with God. There is a story of how, during a period when the sales in the Arya Vaidya Sala dropped sharply, he went to the temple, laid the keys of the Vaidya Sala at the shrine and prostrated, saying to Vishvambharan, 'I leave everything to you.' The next day, there was a large order from Singapore for medicines.

Varier did not believe that tradition should freeze learning or prohibit innovation. His outlook on Ayurveda was therefore critical; he realized that old attitudes had to be discarded and new ones adopted if Ayurveda was to keep pace with a changing world. Once he was in a position to carry out his own decisions, he wasted no time in giving a pragmatic expression to this attitude. The establishment of the Arya Vaidya Sala and the Patasala and the stages in their progress testify to his preoccupation with innovative ideas.

Varier did not involve himself directly in political activities although he maintained an active interest in national and world affairs. N.V. Krishnankutty Warrier, the Ayurvedic scholar, recalls going to receive the Onappudava (a gift of new clothes for the Onam festival) from Varier at the period when he was an enthusiastic young worker for the nationalist cause. To his surprise, he was given khadi mundus. Varier said to him: 'I share your feelings. But it is through my dedication to Ayurveda that I work for my country.'

P.K. Warrier, the present managing trustee, left home and his studies in the Ayurvedic college in 1942 to take part in the

Independence movement. P.S. Varier insisted it was not necessary to send anyone after him or ask him to come back, that he was certain to do so on his own. Sure enough, the young P.K. Warrier did return in two years.

P.S. Varier was undoubtedly a visionary, but he was also extremely practical in his dealings with men and matters; he could be extravagantly generous with money, but he always knew, at every moment, how much he could afford to spend; he expected efficiency and obedience from his subordinates but was scrupulously attentive to their most trivial personal needs. People who met him remembered him for many different qualities: for his wit and scholarship, his musical talent, his administrative capacities, his financial acumen. More than any of these, for his unfailing kindness and generosity.

18

The P.S.V. Natya Sangham

From 1925, with the advent of the cinema, interest in drama gradually began to wane. Well before this, however, P.S. Varier had realized that the time had come to try something more sophisticated than drama, some traditional art with a different and more attractive dimension. He first considered a completely novel idea: why not, he thought, make Koodiyattam, an ancient form of classical dance that could be seen and enjoyed only in the temples, available to audiences everywhere? As early as 1921, he discussed this with the great Koodiyattam maestro, Mani Madhava Chakyar. The artist paid Varier a visit while he was at Kottakkal, performing under the auspices of the kovilakam for the annual festival at the Venkitta Thevar temple. Madhava Chakyar confesses with regret that he was not open at the time to the advantages of this innovative idea:

> We talked about many things and spoke at great length about Koothu and Koodiyattam. Then Varier asked me, 'Will you perform Koodiyattam here, in my hall? If you will, we can start straightaway. In this way, we can give Sanskrit plays a new form of presentation, a

fresh vitality and also take Koodiyattam to many places. After all, we cannot take our temples with us wherever we go. If you are prepared to do this, we can make my drama company and your Sanskrit theatre a single organization. Think it over carefully and tell me,' Varier said. But my situation at that time, the halo of aristocracy that Koodiyattam wore, the narrowness of my own mind, none of these would permit me to accept his suggestion. My attitude later engendered in me a sense of remorse so deep that it still continues to grow.[25]

So the moment when Koodiyattam might have been chosen went by and Varier began to explore other avenues.

The next experiment P.S. Varier tried was to have his actors specially trained to present episodes from the *Mahabharatham* in a style evocative of Kathakali. He chose songs from the repertoire of Kathakali, well-known lyrics written by Irayimman Thambi and Unnayi Varier. Kuthanoor Karunakara Panikker, a reputed actor of the period, particularly skilled at playing women's roles, was engaged to teach the men who played the women's roles in these plays special dances in the slow, sensuous 'lasya' style. But plays of this kind, that belonged neither to the drama nor the Kathakali tradition, failed to please audiences. Sensing that the power of drama was dying and knowing that he had to make a radical change before it was too late, Varier decided to make his drama troupe a full-fledged Kathakali troupe.

The P.S.V. Natya Sangham came into being in 1939. On 16 November 1939, P.S. Varier records in his diary the arrival of cartloads of colourful accessories for the troupe. Thanks to

---

[25]Mani Madhava Chakyar, P. 'Koothunrittam' (The Koothu Dance Form), *Souvenir of Vaidyaratnam P.S. Varier's Centenary Celebrations*, Mathrubhumi Press, p.127-28.

the Kerala Kalamandalam, established by the poet Vallathol Narayana Menon in 1930, there had been a resurgence in the art of Kathakali which had kindled the interest of audiences in Kerala. Many of the members of Varier's drama troupe moved to the Natya Sangham and began their training in Kathakali with the novices. Those who could not move in this way were given other jobs in the Vaidya Sala. It was at this juncture that actor-vaidyans like A.C. Achuthan Nair and Gopi Nedungadi became full-fledged vaidyans and gave up theatre for good.

The first Kathakali performance took place on 25 January 1940. Varier notes the event next morning in his diary:

26 January 1940

The first performance of the Kathakali troupe took place—all went off auspiciously.

Varier was determined to make this Kathakali troupe the best in Kerala. He spared no efforts to get excellent teachers, like Pattikkanthodi Ravunni Menon and his student, K.R. Kumaran. In the very early stages, Guru Kunju Kurup, one of Kerala's most renowned Kathakali teachers, and Kavalappara Narayanan Nair also taught at Kottakkal. One of Ravunni Menon's greatest disciples, Vazhankata Kunju Nair, taught the troupe from 1945 to 1962. Venkatakrishna Bhagavathar, a well-known Kathakali musician of the period, spent a few months at Kottakkal coaching the troupe. His disciple's disciple taught the troupe from 1940 to 1945. Moothamana Namboodiri taught the chenda and Venkatachalaswamy the maddalam. Kadathanattu Sankara Varier was appointed to teach the artistes Sanskrit.

Students who came to learn the different aspects of Kathakali—dance, music, the chenda and the maddalam (the percussion instruments used in Kathakali) and the special make-up for the dancers that is known as 'chutti'—were paid a stipend while they studied. Dance and music took eight years to qualify in, the chenda and maddalam took four years and the chutti, including the making of the accessories, took three years. Those who learned dance had to get up at four in the morning to practise their eye, foot and body exercises. From eight-thirty to twelve and from three to five-thirty they practised cholliyattam, expressing the words of the songs in dance movements to the accompaniment of music. From seven-thirty to nine in the evenings, they learnt Kathakali mudras. Whenever they had time in between all these activities, they studied literature—mainly the poetry that was the life of Kathakali. Those who were learning to sing or play instruments also had to get up at four and practise. Most of the students who learnt with the Natya Sangham found jobs with it when they finished. Others found employment with other troupes.

Kottakkal Krishnankutty Nair, born in 1928, was one of those who moved from the drama troupe to the Kathakali Sangham. He grew up in poverty in a small village called Vadanamkurissi. His relative, E. Sankunni Nair, a distant uncle who worked in Varier's drama troupe, brought him to Kottakkal when he was ten, hoping to find him something to do.

The boy was stunned when he first saw Kailasamandiram: it seemed to him a marvel, like a palace in a mythological tale. More was to follow: he saw an unforgettable play, *Bhakta Nandanar*, in which the electric lights on stage created magical effects. A.C. Achuthan Nair played a most moving Nandanar and the whole play with its gorgeous backdrops, which included the splendid temple of Chidambaram, captivated the child completely.

The next morning, his uncle took him upstairs to P.S. Varier's sumptuous sitting room in Kailasamandiram. A harmonium was tuned and the child was asked to sing. Caught in a web of enchantment, the child sang loudly and untunefully, oblivious to pitch and rhythm. Varier interrupted him and cried out: 'Stop! Stop!' The unfortunate Krishnankutty not only had to go down with his uncle feeling distressed and humiliated, he was also scolded for his failure.

The next day, Varier gave orders for the boy to go on the stage as part of a group of cowherds in the *Krishna Leela*. Feeling slightly relieved but still quite nervous, he managed to do whatever he was told. The following day, he was told that his birthday was the same as the death anniversary of C.P. Kuttikrishnan, the player of women's roles, who had died a few years back. Because of this, his uncle told him, he was considered an incarnation of Kuttikrishnan, and would be taken on in the troupe. Krishnankutty soon vindicated himself and became a talented player of young boys' roles. When the Kathakali troupe was started, he was selected to train in it.

Krishnankutty Nair writes[26] in his reminiscences of how he used to watch P.S. Varier go to the Kathakali hall in the mornings, after he had worshipped in the temple and examined the patients who had been waiting for him. Varier would watch the artistes practise movements to music and then conduct a class for the teachers on how to express ideas in dance movements. If there were padams or slokams in Sanskrit that the teachers wanted explained, he would clear their doubts. He would then help them to find ragas suited to the mood of the songs they had to sing and make them sing. Sometimes, instead of working with them in the practice-hall, Varier would take them upstairs to his room in Kailasamandiram and explain Sanskrit verses to them. Then, with the harmonium tuned to the desired pitch, he would make everyone sing: all the teachers, of music as well as of other subjects, the students and even Shoolapani Varier, the manager. Varier particularly loved the songs in the four days' performance of the *Nala*

---

[26]Krishnankutty Nair: *Ente Adyakaala Jeevithathilekku Oru Thirinjunottam*. (A Backward Glance at My Early Life) Handwritten manuscript lent to me by Krishnankutty Nair.

Charitham, a demanding item and a favourite with him. He would elucidate the difficult Sanskrit words and ask the dancers to demonstrate the appropriate mudras for each word. Krishnankutty Nair acknowledges the extensive help Varier gave him in this way as 'the main reason for successful development in my Kathakali career.'

Until Varier's death, the troupe occasionally performed plays from the old repertoire of drama. After his death, the Kathakali troupe was disbanded for a while, but returned to work after six months and continues to be active in training students and staging performances. It is now one of the most important troupes in Kerala.

The Kathakali performances took place in the temple courtyard at night. Since Varier wanted more and more people to appreciate Kathakali, he also arranged special evening performances once a week between seven and ten in the drama hall, on Saturdays, the day of the Kottakkal weekly market. Crowds of people from neighbouring villages who had come to buy or sell in the market flocked to these performances.

Apart from these regular performances, Varier would sometimes suddenly ask the troupe to perform a particular story, either because he had a guest whom he wanted to entertain, or for his own pleasure. T.P. Rama Pisharoty (known as Kunjan Pisharoty), who had multiple skills—he could dance, sing, play the maddalam or the chengala—acquired a special ability to arrange these instant performances. M. Krishnan Nair would do the chutti for the actors. Ramatharakan, an employee in the factory who was good at costumes, would come hurrying as soon as he was sent for. The man who washed the Kathakali costumes and an Arya Vaidya Sala employee named Kuttikrishnan Nair would hold up the thirasheela, the curtain.

There are frequent diary entries in which Varier records which story his troupe performed on a particular day. In the entries for 28 and 29 August 1941, he gives a complete list of all the stories the troupe had learnt until then—altogether, they number thirty.

Around 1935, Varier constructed a large hall on the southern side of Kailasamandiram, near the Vishvambhara temple, for the Kathakali performers to practise in. A year or two later, when a group of workers came to construct the Puthur bridge near Kottakkal, he hired them to lay a concrete terraced roof over this hall. Concrete was then a novelty. Called the outhouse, this structure has since been considerably modified and extended and is now the residence of the managing trustee.

The members of the troupe ate in Kailasamandiram and Varier was very particular that they be served good food. Once, when the price of coconut oil went up, a decision was taken without consulting Varier to stop frying pappadams for the actors. Varier was very annoyed when he found out. He made no comments, but he refused pappadams when the cook served them for his lunch, giving no reason. When pressed to say why he had refused, he said he did not want to eat anything his employees were denied. The troupe was served pappadams as usual from the next meal.

Kottakkal Krishnankutty Nair speaks[27] of how P.S. Varier's friend, Ambi Iyer, who came for all the Kathakali performances, became a favourite with the actors, especially the younger ones, because he distributed coins to all of them as gifts. If, on one day, he did not have enough coins for everyone, he would give away whatever he had in his pocket, then go to the green room and promise to bring them all a coin each later. He never broke his word: he would calculate how many performers there were and bring the coins next morning. He came to visit Varier every day and the villagers used to say that neither could live without seeing the other.

[27]Ibid.

T. Sankarankutty Nair, one of the principal Kathakali actors, was in trouble once—his chutti, the white beard-like piece around his chin, made of flour and lime-paste, fell off as soon as he stood up. The chutti is applied on the actor's face while he lies flat on the ground. Sankarankutty Nair lay down again and the chutti was redone, with fresh flour. But the moment he got up, it fell off again. This happened quite a few times and, in despair, Sankarankutty Nair sought Varier's help. Varier came to the green room and sat down near Sankarankutty Nair, his hand gently touching him, while his chutti was being done. When it was over, he asked the actor to get up. The chutti stayed in place until the end of the evening.

A Muslim employee in the Arya Vaidya Sala named Thenu used to measure medicines and fill them in tins that he welded himself. Varier asked him to think about a new way to make chuttis which normally took a long time to apply: the paccha, the one painted green, for a good character took two and a half hours, a kathi for a base character with a knife-shaped moustache took almost four hours. Thenu decided to try a tin sheet instead of flour and lime-paste. He cut it in shape, painted it with rice flour and secured it firmly to the actor's chin and behind his ears with rubber bands. Varier was very pleased when he saw this invention since he was always looking for ways to save time on the make-up for the Kathakali artistes. He asked Thenu to make chuttis for all the actors. It saved them so much time that when other troupes saw the chuttis, they wanted them made too. These tin chuttis fell into disuse only when light ones made of paper came into vogue.

P.S. Varier used the electrical devices he had invented for drama in Kathakali as well, to make the scenes more attractive to spectators. For example, there were props to simulate an illuminated garden in the *Nala Charitham*; when Ravanan sang to the full moon in the *Toranayuddham*, it appeared above him.

Varier used to love standing upstairs in Kailasamandiram, watching the children of the drama and Kathakali troupes play in the temple yard. Sometimes he would ask the man who looked after his elephant, Balan, to bring the elephant to the yard and give each of the children a ride. There were occasions when the children playing in the yard would be surprised to see a sudden shower of oranges rain over their heads and bounce over the ground. They would look up to see Varier at the window, signing to them to catch the fruit as it fell!

Mekkara Narayanan Nair,[28] who joined the P.S.V. Natya Sangham in 1942 met Varier only once, but has an unforgettable story to relate about his career in the troupe.

Narayanan had worked as a child with a Kathakali troupe in Kannur, doing the chutti for the dancers. His older brother had been in this troupe and run away, and their uncle had brought young Narayanan to make up for his brother's rash behaviour. The child had not even been to school. The troupe's owner, Nayanar, kept animals for his amusement— monkeys, elephants and peacocks and the child enjoyed running around the vast compound, watching them. He was gradually trained to make and apply chuttis.

He first visited Kottakkal with Nayanar's troupe in 1941 and made friends with the young boys in the P.S.V. Natya Sangham. Being the youngest, he was treated with great affection by both troupes. He enjoyed his stay at Kottakkal, the ambience of Kailasamandiram, the excellent food, his lively companions. Shortly after he returned to Kannur, Nayanar died and the troupe was disbanded. Narayanan stayed at home for a while, not sure what to do. He had no education and making chuttis was the only skill he had acquired. Recalling the pleasant time

---

[28]I am indebted for the details of this story to Mekkara Narayanan Nair himself. He narrated it to me when I met him at Kottakkal in 1999.

he had spent at Kottakkal, he decided to go there to seek a livelihood. He somehow made his way from Payyannur to Kottakkal, walking, begging rides for part of the way. The younger Kathakali dancers at Kottakkal remembered him and advised him to go to Rama Pisharoty, who was actually in charge of the Kathakali performances. Shoolapani Varier continued to be the manager of the troupe, but he had still not learnt enough about Kathakali, he knew much more about drama. The Kottakkal boys felt that he might not allow Narayanan to stay.

Rama Pisharoty asked the boy what he could do and gave him permission to stay with them for a while. A couple of days later, he asked Narayanan to do a chutti to test his skill. It was work the boy was familiar with, he did it faster and better than the old man who worked with the troupe and much more effortlessly, eager to finish it and go away to play! Rama Pisharoty was impressed. The boy evidently knew his job and his eyes were sharper than the old man's, a distinct advantage when working on a chutti.

Rama Pisharoty told Varier about the boy and Narayanan was asked to make chuttis for the entire troupe from the next day at a salary of a rupee a month—a sum of money he never actually saw, since Sankunni Nair, the odd-job man of the troupe, took all the children's salaries for himself. But the boy did not care—he was happy doing what he did. The food served in the northern wing of Kailasamandiram was good and plentiful. Rice, four kinds of vegetable preparations, pappadams. Four mundus a year, two towels, two jubbas. Friends, playmates, long periods of time for play between performances. What more could he ask for?

Narayanan often used to see Varier at a distance, going into the temple or walking through the village in the evening or teaching the musicians and dancers in the Kathakali troupe but not once did the boy dare approach or speak to him.

3

Six months passed and Narayanan wanted to visit his home. His request was conveyed to Varier, who instructed the manager to give the boy twenty-five rupees for the journey. The manager suggested that Narayanan keep five rupees with him and the rest be sent as a money order to his home in Payyanur. Narayanan was hurt. 'Surely I know how to take care of my money. I'll keep all of it with me,' he insisted.

So he set out by bus with a little box, his money in a small purse tucked into the pocket of his jubba and a letter to the Jamalia Press in Tirur containing instructions to buy him a ticket to Payyanur. At Tirur, he boarded the train for Payyannur. When the train stopped at the Kozhikode station, he caught sight of a basket of oranges and wanted to buy one, but found his purse missing! He wept loudly, feeling utterly bereft. He had no ticket and no money, he knew no one in Kozhikode, what would he do? Fellow passengers asked him from where he had come and a kindly man offered to take him to the Arya Vaidya Sala in Kozhikode. Narayanan told the people at the Arya Vaidya Sala his sorry tale. He was given a meal and told to wait while a letter was sent by the bus which went from Kozhikode to Kottakkal. The reply came back on the same bus: if Narayanan wants to go home, buy him a ticket to Payyanur. If he wants to come back to Kottakkal, send him on the bus.

The boy chose to go home. He was given twenty rupees and his ticket. This time, he tucked the money securely into his waist, fastened a towel tightly around it, folded his mundu above his knees and tucked the ends around the towel. He arrived home safe and returned to Kottakkal in a week.

To his surprise, when he got back to Kottakkal, he received a money order for five rupees, signed by P.S. Varier himself. Narayanan had originally been given twenty-five rupees and the Kozhikode Arya Vaidya Sala had given him only twenty. Varier had found this out and sent the remaining five

rupees to Payyanur, from where it had been redirected to
Kottakkal since the boy had left by the time it arrived.
Overwhelmed by the generosity of a person who had
remembered even this small detail, Narayanan put away the
money order receipt safely, a precious souvenir of his escapade,
with no idea that it was going to stand him in good stead on
a later occasion.

He was also summoned to appear before Varier. He went
up the stairs in Kailasamandiram, quaking with fear, knees
knocking. All Varier said was, 'Little idiot! Imagine putting
your purse in the pocket of your jubba like that! Run off now.'

It was the only time Narayanan met P.S. Varier, but he
still carries with him the memory of an extraordinary concern
and generosity, the realization that this man who had so much
to attend to every day, so many people working under him
whose affairs he looked after, could still remember and
acknowledge the services of a small boy who did the chuttis for
his Kathakali dancers.

But it did not end with that. After Varier's death, the
Kathakali troupe dispersed for some months, until a decision
could be taken about their future. Many of them were actually
recalled within the year. Unfortunately, Narayanan was away
from home, working somewhere else, when the letter asking
him to go back to Kottakkal arrived at his house. It took a
while for his old friends to trace him and tell him to come
back to Kottakkal. When he finally rejoined, there had been a
gap of about two years in his service.

At the time of his retirement, this gap in service presented
an obstacle to his receiving a pension. How could he prove
that he had been with the troupe from 1942 to 1944, before
P.S. Varier's death, they asked. Narayanan suddenly recalled
the saga of his first trip home and produced the money order
receipt of 1942, signed by Varier. What further proof did the
authorities need?

Mekkara Narayanan Nair learnt how to read and write after he joined the Kathakali troupe in Kottakkal. He recalls that one of his great pleasures in life was being able to read and enjoy the Malayalam translation of Jawaharlal Nehru's *Discovery of India*. He has no doubts at all that he and his entire family owe everything they have to P.S. Varier. That, thanks to Varier's abiding concern for the welfare of his employees, all of them have lived and are still able to live, in reasonable comfort and security.

19

The Will

Early in life, P.S. Varier had learnt from his mother that whatever he earned by his own efforts had to be kept separate from the wealth and property that belonged to the family, the taravad. The feeling that not all his family members supported him in this became a source of worry to him as he grew older and his establishments stabilized. One of the factors that led him to make a will was his anxiety to adhere to this distinction. The terms of the will were altered three times and it is believed that he wanted to make some more changes just before he died, but that death took him away before he did so.

The main thrust of the will he drafted was directed towards the administration of the establishments he had founded. For this, he selected a trust board composed of reliable and capable people from among members of his family and people connected to the Arya Vaidya Sala. He had to make the manner in which he wanted them to manage the affairs of each establishment clear to them. He evidently wanted to make a few more changes in the third will written in 1939 and had discussed them with a close friend on 28 January 1944 and asked him to arrange for a lawyer to come from Palakkad on 30 January to draft another document. But he died very early on the morning of the thirtieth, and that will was never written. It was the document he had registered in 1939 that took effect after his death.

The second clause of this will of 1939 deals with the distinction Varier draws between his family possessions and his own, his own being the income he received from the establishments he had founded with his personal earnings:

2. The properties shown in Schedule A belong to my taravad and include items the taravad originally possessed as well as those which I acquired and gave to the taravad. Barring the items shown in this schedule, all other properties, movable as well as immovable, and all other outstandings and transactions standing in my name, the institutions known as the Arya Vaidya Sala, the Arya Vaidya Hospital and allied institutions together with all outstandings relating to them are my private possessions acquired through personal effort without recourse to or detriment to the taravad properties and I have full powers of disposition over them. Apart from the properties in Schedule A, there are no other taravad properties in my possession.

In the fourth and fifth clauses, he handed over certain portions of this private wealth that he had amassed by his own efforts to his Cheriyamma, Kutty Varasyar's two surviving daughters, Lakshmi Varasyar and Kunji Varasyar and their respective families. Since, according to the matrilinear system, these are actually the same family, the name used in Malayalam to distinguish one branch from another is 'tavazhi'. Kutty Varasyar, P.S. Varier's Cheriyamma, and her children had been the only immediate family that Varier could claim as his own for many years now. Varier had already made provision for his

Cheriyamma's son, P.V. Krishna Varier in 1941, when he signed the document relieving him of his family responsibilities.

The sixth clause deals with the administration of the Vishvambhara temple, which was to be handed over to the two tavazhis mentioned in the fourth and fifth clauses, those of Lakshmi Varasyar and Kunji Varasyar. Varier describes the temple as a shrine that he installed so that he and the members of his family could worship there. He had funded its expenditure with his own earnings and wished this to continue. Each tavazhi was therefore to be in charge of conducting all the rituals and ceremonies for a whole year, the other tavazhi was to take over the next year. They were each to spend a sum of not less than six hundred rupees every year on carrying out these duties. If one tavazhi were to fail in doing so, the other had to take over, have the ceremonies performed and recover the money they had spent from the defaulters. If both defaulted, the trustees had to collect the required amounts of money from the properties of the two tavazhis and perform the ceremonies themselves. Not more than one per cent of the amount realized from the sale of medicines in the Arya Vaidya Sala was to be used for extraordinary expenses for the temple; in this way, the activities of the temple would also serve as a means of publicity for the Vaidya Sala. Varier thus engaged the involvement of his family members as well as of the trustees in the administration of the temple. By 1944, the annual festival had become a well-known feature, a phenomenon that attracted spectators from far and near since, besides the processions and rituals, there were cultural programmes of a high order on every day of the festival. This meant that Varier had already ensured the element of publicity, an aspect that the trustees were sure to appreciate and respect.

The seventh clause stated that all the remaining properties would go to a trust which would be administered by a board of trustees and went on to name the trustees. They were seven in number:

I hereby nominate the following persons as the first board of trustees.

Rao Bahadur Dr Pulakkat Krishna Varier, L.M.S. Nellaya, Walluvanad.

Dr Pulakkat Ramankutty Warrier, L.M.P. Nellaya, Walluvanad.

Deshamangalath Wariath Rama Warrier, Vyakaranasiromani, Talapalli Taluk, Deshamangalath Village.

Cherunellikkat Wariath Rama Warrier, Marakkara.

Aryavaidyan P. Madhava Warrier, Kottakkal.

Aryavaidyan P.V. Rama Varier, Manager, Arya Vaidya Sala Branch, Kozhikode.

Thenkurissi Krishna Menon, Head Clerk, Arya Vaidya Sala, Kottakkal.

All the trustees were to hold office for life unless they resigned. The first five were part of the family and belonged to the two tavazhis mentioned earlier. Pulakkat Krishna Varier was Lakshmi Varasyar's son-in-law and Pulakkat Rama Warrier her grandson-in-law; Deshamangalath Wariath Rama Warrier and Cherunellikkat Wariath Rama Warrier were Parvathy (Kunji) Varasyar's sons-in-law. Aryavaidyan P. Madhava Warrier was Kunji Varasyar's son and P.S. Varier's direct nephew. Aryavaidyan P.V. Rama Varier had been P.S. Varier's student and later his trusted assistant, the physician in charge of the branch at Kozhikode. Shinnan Menon had been the head clerk at the Arya Vaidya Sala from the time it was started and one of the most reliable members of Varier's staff.

P. Madhava Warrier, P.S. Varier's nephew, was appointed the first managing trustee. The managing trustee had to preside over the meetings of the board of trustees. All decisions were to be taken according to the opinion of the majority and the managing trustee had, besides his own vote, a casting vote. Madhava Warrier was to hold office for life, but, if for some reason, he ceased to be the managing trustee, the board had to choose a new person from among themselves and, as far as possible, this had to be a member belonging to one of the two tavazhis who were represented on the trust. The new incumbent could then hold office for five years, at the end of which there was to be a fresh nomination for which he too would be eligible.

The trust was to carry out all the objectives of the Arya Vaidya Sala and the Arya Vaidya Chikitsasala with a view to enlarging their range and scope and their usefulness to the public on the lines that Varier had already marked out for them. The will specified these objectives clearly. The Vaidya Sala's was to process and sell Ayurvedic medicines; to treat patients and receive from them compensation in keeping with their means; to conduct the kind of research into aryavaidyam that would increase its usefulness to the public. The hospital had to examine poor patients who came to the out-patient wing free of charge, prescribe treatment and give them free medicines; to take in at least twelve poor patients at a time, provide board, lodging, medicines and treatment free for them as in-patients; to carry out these services with the help of an aryavaidyan and perform surgical procedures if necessary with the help of a doctor trained in western medicine; to give medicines and treatment to all who sought them, receiving from them only what each of them could afford to give for these services.

The will went on to state how the profits from the Arya Vaidya Patasala were to be used:

L. Out of the net profits of the Arya Vaidya Sala, 25% is to be devoted to the development of the Arya Vaidya Sala, 25% for meeting the expenses of the Arya Vaidya Hospital and 25% for equal division between the two tavazhis (this only for 20 years). Out of the remaining 25%, a sum not exceeding 10% may be, according to requirements, utilized for the purposes of the Arya Vaidya Patasala. The balance, if any, that may remain out of the 10% after disbursement to the Arya Vaidya Patasala may be used for the Arya Vaidya Sala itself. The remaining 15% is to be deposited by the trustees each year in approved banks as a reserve fund for the two tavazhis for a period of 20 years and the fund thus accumulated inclusive of interest is to be divided equally between the two tavazhis i.e. in moiety and it will be the duty of the trustees to invest the same on the security of immovable properties.

M. The trustees are not bound to pay any amount to the said two tavazhis after the expiry of 20 years. 40% of the profits so earmarked for 20 years and so released after the expiry of 20 years is thereafter to be utilized for the development of the Arya Vaidya Sala and the Arya Vaidya Hospital according to the discretion of the trustees.

This distribution of the profits earned from enterprises that were wholly Varier's own effort shows a rare impartiality and a remarkable insight into the needs of each of the beneficiaries he mentions. The Arya Vaidya Sala was always uppermost in P.S. Varier's mind: it was the most unique of his establishments, something that he had conceived and realized as an answer to an urgent need. Also, it was for him the best, the most efficient way to propagate Ayurveda, to make it available to everyone, rich or poor. Therefore the continued development of all its facets was an important activity for the progress of Ayurveda and he wanted to make certain that it would not lack the funds for expansion. The provision he made for his nieces and their children had a double purpose: it ensured their comfort for twenty years after his death. And in those twenty years, he expected them to prosper, to become self-sufficient enough to be able to attend to their own welfare without help from him.

The next clause was to do with Kailasamandiram:

> The building known as Kailasamandiram mentioned in E Schedule is not intended for the use of patients. The managing trustee and such of the trustees as are related to the two tavazhis mentioned in para 4 are entitled to reside therein according to the decision of the trust board. Further, the trustees are to provide temporary residence, necessary amenities to guests who visit in connection with the affairs of the Arya Vaidya Sala.

The trustees were to continue to run the Parama Shiva Vilasam Nataka Company (it had not yet become the P.S.V. Natya Sangham Kathakali troupe when the will of 1939 was written) even if it inflicted minimal losses on them, since it would serve as a means of publicity for the Arya Vaidya Sala. However, the trustees could disband it if they felt it was necessary to do so. In this case, equipment like curtains, props and musical instruments were to be given to the ten people who had the longest service in the troupe.

Pensions were to be given to all who had completed thirty years of service in the Arya Vaidya Sala at the time of P.S. Varier's death, at the rate usually allowed for government servants. If there were sufficient funds and if the trustees felt it was necessary, pensions or gratuities could be given to other employees who retired at a later date after thirty years of service. P.S. Varier had always evinced deep concern for his employees and this clause, conceived at a time when pensions were hardly thought of as compulsory, when the main concern of people who ran private establishments was to somehow make money for themselves, was unusually far-sighted and generous.

Varier set apart a sum that was not to exceed Rs 10,000 from the assets of the Arya Vaidya Sala for his funeral expenses and between Rs 200 to 300 for his annual shraddha ceremony and the tila homam (a sacrificial offering with sesame seeds) and poor feeding which he performed every year on the anniversary of his mother's death.

Varier recorded registering the will of 1939 on 15 February 1940 in his diary.

In 1941, all the members of the Panniyinpally family signed a document that relieved Varier of the entire responsibilities of the taravad and left him free to do what he wanted with regard to the administration of the Arya Vaidya Sala and the Patasala. The diary entry of 15 April 1941 records their having signed this document and speaks of the period for which he held the post of the karanavar, the seniormost male member of the taravad:

15 April 1941

It is 35 years, 7 months and 8 days since Amma died. I have held the post of karanavar for 60 years and 4 months.

10 July 1941

The family document was registered today, 1–201 of 1941, no.1145-7

In the diary entry for 20 June 1941, Varier wrote that he divided the family jewels among the members of the family. There are two small entries on either side of the date, each mentioning a list: a vairaminni (a diamond necklace) and an ilakkathali (a gold necklace) are common to both; he mentions that each list is for one tavazhi, the two main branches of the family.

20 June 1941

Divided the taravad jewels. Kept only Amma's bangles.

The same year, 1941, he gifted properties worth more than seven thousand rupees to his cousin P.V. Krishna Varier's family.

What further changes Varier wanted to make in this remarkable document is something we will never know. Since the Parama Shiva Vilasam Nataka Company had become a Kathakali troupe from 1939, it is almost certain that he would have wanted to make changes relevant to the dispersal of the old troupe and the formation of the new one. But even as it stands now, the will shows a perception and farsightedness that are exceptional, a true comprehension of what it meant to establish a business concern that consistently aimed at the welfare of all, not of one person or his immediate family.

The profits the Arya Vaidya Sala have continued to earn prove beyond any doubt that P.S. Varier's decision to channel them back into measures for its growth and development was remarkably astute. The turnover at the time of his death in 1944 was Rs 3.3 lakh. It has since increased to Rs 7.5 lakh in 1950, Rs 213.1 lakh in 1975 and Rs 5999.4 lakh in 2000.

20

Turning Seventy

These were hard times. The Second World War was going on. P.S. Varier had been following the course of the war closely:

3 September 1939

Britain and Germany have declared war on each other.

28 October 1940

Italy attacked Greece early morning today.

8 December 1941

Japan has declared war on Britain and America and launched an attack. Singapore is affected as well.

Varier had cause to be particularly concerned about Singapore since the Arya Vaidya Sala regularly sent a large quantity of medicines to that country.

It was twenty-five years since the Patasala had been established and Varier was anxious to celebrate the occasion. But many of his friends and well-wishers wondered whether it was fitting to conduct celebrations of any kind during this grim period. Varier held firmly to his decision. 'I am seventy-two,' he declared. 'I celebrated the Silver Jubilee of the Arya Vaidya Sala in a very grand manner. I cannot allow the Silver Jubilee of the Patasala to go unnoticed while I am alive.'

The jubilee celebrations took place as Varier wished on 24 and 25 January 1942. They started with a colourful procession with elephants and percussion at three-thirty on the afternoon of the 24th. In the evening, there was an exhibition of herbs followed by the production of the play, *Naishadham*.

On 25 January, the second day, a report was read on the Patasala and an oil painting of Vaidyaratnam P.S. Varier was unveiled. The students, old and new, presented an address to Varier. Diplomas were given during the afternoon session, after which there were speeches by guest speakers. A tea party followed. There was an all-night Kathakali performance of the *Nala Charitham* which Varier attended. Kalamandalam Krishnan Nair one of the most distinguished artistes of Vallathol's Kerala Kalamandalam came for this performance.

A souvenir was released on the occasion. Besides numerous articles in Malayalam, Sanskrit and English on many aspects of vaidyam by well-known vaidyans, it contained the names of all the students who had qualified from the Patasala from 1921 to 1941 and the photographs of some of the more distinguished diploma holders, including that of Aryavaidya A. Ammukutty Amma, the first woman to take her diploma, in 1934. The volume also included a list of the most important herbs and exhibits displayed at the exhibition organized for the occasion with their names listed in Malayalam, Sanskrit and Latin or English.

Among the many advertisements in the souvenir was a full-page one for the products of the Arya Vaidya Sala, Kottakkal, giving the names of certain preparations, their dosage, price and the indication for their use.

Varier resumed the writing of the *Brihadshareeram* that he

had abandoned years earlier and was able to release the first part during the Silver Jubilee function. The second part remained incomplete. The manuscript was put together after his death and the second part was published in 1969, on the occasion of his birth centenary.

Over the years, the patients who came to the Charitable Hospital had come to attribute a healing touch to their 'Varierachan' (Father Varier) as they called him affectionately. Local legends took shape about the powers of this touch.

One of these legends feature Ambi Iyer who had an unforgettable experience that gave him one more excellent reason to value Varier's friendship. Varier saved him on this occasion from certain death. Ambi Iyer had a strangulated hernia for which he had tried all kinds of remedies with no success. Desperate with pain one night, he sent for a doctor who advised him to go as soon as he could to Kozhikode for surgery. Sure that he would never come back alive, Ambi Iyer insisted that he had to see Varier before he left Kottakkal. It was already very late at night and his family was worried: how could they disturb Varier at that hour? Finally, they sent for their relative, Shinnan Menon, who agreed to go and explain the emergency to Varier. Varier made ready to go to Ambi Iyer at once. As he hurried out, he picked up a small bottle that was on his table and took it with him.

When Varier entered his room, Ambi was in tears. 'I had to see you, I will soon be gone. My children are still young, you must look after them,' he lamented. Varier laid Ambi's head on his lap and comforted him. 'No, no, you're not going anywhere. Who will come with me to watch the temple festival and the Kathakali performances if you go away like that? You'll be all right.' As he spoke, Varier inserted his finger into the bottle he had brought with him and rubbed something on Ambi's tongue. Miraculously, the hernia moved up and settled back, releasing Ambi from the agony he had been enduring for days. Varier sat with him while some kanji was made, made sure he drank it and then left.

S. Varier, who was working in the Palakkad branch at the time this incident took place, was intrigued to hear of it and asked Varier when he next visited the branch, 'What did you rub on Ambi Iyer's tongue?'

'Dhanvantharam 101,' replied Varier. This was a concentrate obtained by processing the medicine repeatedly 101 times. 'Haven't you heard, "moothraghathanthravridhijil?"' he asked. The phrase means that hernia can occur when there are obstacles to passing urine. The drug had obviously released the obstruction.

Ambi Iyer's son, Radhakrishna Menon, had equally convincing experiences to relate.[29] The first was when he was a child. Every summer, he developed an allergic rash on his body. It was accompanied with high fever and itched unbearably. The third summer, his mother asked Ambi Iyer to show the child to Varier. Seated on a servant's shoulder, the little boy was taken up to Varier's room in Kailasamandiram. Varier took a look at him and said, 'It's nothing serious,' prescribed a kashayam and lehyam to be taken internally and asked Ambi to see that the child was given a bath with nalpamaradi thailam, a medicinal oil. Ambi Iyer's wife was worried and nervous: how could the child be given a bath when he was running a high temperature? But Ambi Iyer had no such fears. We have to do whatever Varier asked us to do, he said, so let's go ahead. They gave the child his bath in the courtyard, late in the evening, when it was cool. The fever went down the next morning and after fourteen days' treatment, the rash disappeared as well. It never recurred.

---

[29]Radhakrishna Menon narrated these experiences at a meeting I had with him at his house in Kottakkal in January 2001.

Radhakrishna Menon had a stranger incident to relate about his older brother, who used to work as a Controller of Naval Accounts in Bombay. Every time he came home on leave, he visited Varier to pay his respects to him. Late in 1943, he came as usual to Kòttakkal and went to Kailasamandiram to see Varier. He was a sturdy, well-built man and the picture of good health. He met Varier, spoke to him and was about to leave. Varier suddenly asked, 'You feel all right? There's nothing wrong with you?' 'I feel fine,' said the young man. He returned to Bombay and was back at Kottakkal within the month, feeling very ill, with tuberculosis of the intestine. He died soon after. By the time he came back, however, Varier was no more. Radhakrishna Menon often wondered later whether Varier had seen the signs of impending illness, or even impending death, the morning his brother last visited Kailasamandiram.

Another of Varier's professional successes brought him a valuable piece of land, the one that serves at present as the car park for Kailasamandiram, on the side of the road that runs by the Arya Vaidya Sala. This land originally belonged to the princes of the kovilakam and they were unwilling to sell it. Then the senior thampuran had a paralytic stroke and could not move his hands. He tried courses of treatment recommended by various Ashtavaidyans, with no relief. Ambi Iyer, a constant visitor at the kovilakam, suggested they send for P.S. Varier. The thampuran was dubious. 'He's a man with a great reputation now, will he come if I send for him?' 'Of course he will,' said Ambi Iyer.

Varier's prescription proved efficacious. The thampuran was very happy. But Varier would not accept a fee. The thampuran was anxious to show his appreciation. Ambi Iyer suggested that he give Varier the piece of land in front of Kailasamandiram. In return, the kovilakam requested Varier to give them a small piece of land that he owned so that the

Brahmins in Kottakkal could have a cremation ground of their own.

Although the rasayana treatment had refreshed his health and spirits, Varier no longer felt as strong as he had been ten years earlier. He was concerned about his diabetes and monitored his diet very strictly. Occasional bouts of arthritis had begun to affect him. The time and consideration he had devoted so single-mindedly to the drafting of his will was taking its toll. And an astrological prediction lay at the back of his mind: it had been foretold that his death would take place soon after he turned seventy. He was often heard to remark after his seventieth birthday, half in jest, that the astrologer who had made this prediction was very reliable, that he never made mistakes . . .

P.S. Varier had always had a keen interest in horoscopes. He used to cast his own on the first of every Malayalam month and read the signs. On 17 June 1938, he recorded in his diary the calculation of an extraordinary phenomenon, the precise moment when he was conceived in his mother's womb:

17 June 1938

Thinking about the moment I was conceived in my mother's womb, I see that it occurred on Wednesday, 30 Edavam, which makes the period of pregnancy 278 days, 10 nazhikas (a nazhika is 24 minutes) and 10 vinazhikas (a vinazhika is 1/60th of a nazhika or 24 seconds).

18 June 1938

The night of Wednesday, 30 Edavam, the star is Avittam, the rashi is Kumbham: this is more or less the time of conception.

1940 was a calm year. There are numerous diary entries about the gradual addition of items the new Kathakali troupe made to their repertoire and lists of the members of the troupe. The routine for the year mentions that Varier set apart an hour every morning for working with the troupe.

On 22 and 23 January, the diary notes predictions accompanied by zodiac signs. These notes conclude with the remark that all the astrologers had agreed that a very bad time lay ahead for Varier.

The diaries of 1941 mention documents that obviously concern P.V. Krishna Varier's debts. In entries made on 9 January 1941 and 22 January 1941, P.S. Varier refers to his having refused earlier to clear these debts. Subsequent entries mentioned the numbers of court documents dating back to the years 1926, 1927 and 1931. These entries, made in bolder and more carefully written characters than the usual ones for the day, suggest that these documents and dates were important and probably a source of anxiety to P.S. Varier.

On 9 September 1941, Varier repeats that it is thirty-five years since his mother died. On 15 September, he writes:

15 September 1941

Ravunni Panikker wrote that it is a bad time from the month of Chingam (August–September) to Vrischikam (November–December). Must conduct rituals of propitiation.

On 18 January 1942, Varier composed a verse describing his lamentable position as the erstwhile karanavan of the family:

Karanavasthanam poyi
Kaikaryathinarhanallathayi
Kaivashamuthalum kuravayi
Keerthikkumpakamadhikavum kuravayi
Kevalanayum vannu
Kolam ksheenichu vridhanayitheernu
Kashtathapalathum chernnu
Krishnanullam thelinjeetukil nannu

(My position as the karanavan is gone. Therefore I am no longer worthy enough to carry on the family affairs. My wealth has decreased. I am an old man, my body has weakened. So many problems plague me. Krishna, if you would clear your heart for me . . .)

Clearly, he was beset by many worries throughout 1941. There were the problems of P.V. Krishna Varier's debts and the mention of court documents probably indicates another source of harassment. Although the surrender of his position as the head of the family, had made it easier for him to dispose of the properties in the way he wanted, the diary entries suggest a growing feeling of regret and loss. Perhaps the circumstances that had obliged him to take these steps saddened him, or their finality. Whatever it was, it is certain that the combination of all these worries and of the measures he took to resolve them made him feel suddenly old and bereft of strength.

On 5 November 1941, Varier records having seen a sign that seemed to him a premonition:

5 November 1941

At night, seated at dinner, saw the moon double. Looking carefully, it seemed as if there were five small moons. After dinner, looked again and saw the same thing. A sign of death . . .

On 24 December 1941, the verse on giving up the position of a karanavan is repeated. Physical weakness was beginning to tell on him as much as cares and worries:

22 May 1942

I often cry out, 'Ayyo', 'Aavoo', 'I'm so tired' and so on at night, because of fatigue. Sometimes even in the daytime . . .

But he continued to carry out as many of his duties as he could manage: teaching the students of the Patasala and the members of the Kathakali troupe, involving himself with indefatigable zeal in the affairs of the Arya Vaidya Sala.

And there were always distractions. During the floods of 1942, the fields, the wells, and the tanks on the east and south of Kailasamandiram were completely inundated. The water rose to a level that was just below the steps of the Vishvambhara temple and actually touched the gopuram of the Venkitta Thevar temple to the north, since it lay at a lower level. Krishnankutty Nair, the Kathakali artiste, recalls P.S. Varier circling the area in a boat with Sankunni Nair, T. Sankarankutty Nair, Maramveetil Achuthan Nair, Shoolapani Varier and the car driver Narayanan Nair. Shoolapani Varier rowed, singing boat songs, while the Kathakali students followed in another boat, singing after him, repeating each line.

An epidemic of cholera broke out after the floods and Varier made and distributed special medicines, as he had done in 1902, just after the Arya Vaidya Sala was founded. He persuaded the sick to go on a diet, observe very strict rules of hygiene and take their medicines regularly. He was actually able to prevent many deaths.

Krishnankutty Nair also relates how the Kathakali students, who stayed in the outhouses in Kailasamandiram, found it difficult to go on with their usual routine while cholera raged in the village. But their teacher was unrelenting and had no other thought except the daily exercises and practice so vital for Kathakali performers. Finally, Varier intervened and requested him to slow down these activities for a time. The teacher had to obey, though he did so quite unhappily.

Meanwhile, throughout this period of emotional turmoil, Varier continued to mull over the news from the world outside Kottakkal:

7 August 1941
Rabindranath Tagore died this morning at 12.30.

13 February 1942
Sovereign—price—Rs 35.4.0.

27 April 1942
No current. Black-out.

11 June 1942
Italy proclaimed war last night.

24 June 1942
The French signed a treaty tonight. It seems war ceased
in France on Friday at 5.35.

12 August 1942
Gandhiji and others have been arrested.

15 August 1942
A thousand German planes flew into England. 144 of
them were shot down.

9 September 1942
Today, sovereign in Madras—Rs 42.

14 September 1942
Because sugar is so scarce, everyone will have jaggery
with their coffee.

6 October 1942
Sovereign in Madras—price—Rs 43.8.0.

15 October 1942
Terrible gale and cyclone in Bombay.

22 October 1942
The Germans and the Russians have been fighting in
Russia for more than three months. Such modern
weapons have never been used before.

2 November 1942
Sovereign—price—Rs 46.

10 November 1942
Massive earthquake in Rumania. Great destruction.

There has not been such a terrible earthquake since 1802.

10 February 1943
Mahatma Gandhi is to go on hunger strike for 21 days.

26 March 1943
Sovereign—price—Rs 51

12 October 1943
The Mail is delayed because of floods in Madras.

The figures in the diary continued to indicate that the earnings of the Arya Vaidya Sala that Varier kept aside for an emergency, ready cash that he could count on at any time, had been mounting over these years. They are jotted down at the top corners of the diary entries. They are as high as Rs 70,000 in October 1943; by January 1944, they touch Rs 82,576.

The routine described in the diary of 1943 for the year 1942 showed that, in spite of all his worries, Varier did not relax his general rules of discipline:

Get up before 6, check my pulse. Every five days, check respiration as well and then weight. 6.20, go to the toilet. Clean teeth, try for a motion. Most days, am successful. Check weight after this.

6.45, coffee—1 to 1¼ cups with a snack made of wheat. Rest a little, then write my diary. Go through the letters that came the evening before. Most days the paper would not have come. May have a motion again at 8.30. 9.15—1 to 1¼ cups tea and a little more than half a nenthran banana. Some biscuits, pappadam. 9.30, worship Vishvambharan. Then examine patients, if there are any. Otherwise, go to the Kathakali practice-hall. Go upstairs at 10.15, lie down. Then I write something, or explain meanings of the songs to the Kathakali performers. 11, have a meal of wheat with butter. Generally three servings of the cooked wheat. Green leafy vegetables, ginger, pappadams, boiled buttermilk. After the meal, check my pulse. 11.20, lie down until 2. Most days, sleep for a while. After 2, write replies, 30 to 40 minutes. May sleep a bit after finishing this. 3.30, coffee with roasted raw banana, or jaggery dosa. Read the paper. Lie down again at 4. 5 to 5.30, walk for a while. 6.30, have tea. Write something. Then have an oil bath. 8.30, light meal. No ghee, like in the morning. 9.30, go to bed. Usually have 6 to 7 hours sleep. Most days, Sankarankutty is around to assist me; if he can't come, there's Sridharan or one of the other boys.

On 8 January 1943, he records the quantities of food he restricts himself to:

8 January 1943

2½ ladles of rice, rarely more. Coffee twice a day, 1 cup. Tea, 1¼ cup. Rarely go beyond this.

There is then, over this period, a sense of slowing down, of waiting.

21

At Rest

The annual festival of the Vishvambhara temple in Kottakkal, conducted over seven days, became a cultural event that people in Malabar looked forward to every year. The first seven days, there were splendid processions with caparisoned elephants, accompanied by expert melam players; there were performances every evening that often featured artistes and arts from outside Kerala. Nor did the celebrations end with this seven-day festival, the last day of which was P.S. Varier's birthday. The paattu festivals featuring distinctive Kerala temple arts began on the eighth day: first there was the vettaykkoru makan's paattu in honour of the Hunter's Son, when coconuts were thrown as an offering to the deity by expert throwers to the steady, mounting beats of chendas. Then came the Ayyappan paattu, an offering of lamps and songs dedicated to the god Ayyappan, after which there was the Bhagavathi paattu for the Goddess. Crowds came from outside Kottakkal to see, hear and worship.

As the years progressed and he began to experience the satisfaction of realizing a particular goal he had set himself,

Varier began to take particular delight in vowing a special offering to demonstrate his gratitude to the gods. Of these offerings, the one he favoured most was the paattu offering for the vettaykkoru makan, the offering of coconuts to the beautiful son born to Shiva and Parvathy when they once went hunting in the forest. Varier had conducted this offering many times, each occasion marking a point of success. The offering of 12,000 coconuts he vowed to make on 29 December 1943 was to assume a special significance not only for him but for all the people who were present that day in the temple.

While going for a drive in the car that evening P.S. Varier said to Aryavaidyan S. Varier,[30] his one-time student and a trusted disciple,

> When I established the Vaidya Sala, I had no extravagant desires. I thought I would be satisfied if I could make a profit of a rupee a day above what I had spent on it. It did not take me long to reach that stage. And then ... isn't it human nature, after all? As the prosperity of the Arya Vaidya Sala grew, so did my ambitions for it. If I sell medicines for Rs 12,000 a month, I thought, I will have twelve thousand coconuts broken at a vettaykkoru makan paattu. And when I achieved that, I vowed to offer another twelve thousand coconuts if I made Rs 12,000 a month on the sales of medicines at the head office of the Arya Vaidya Sala at Kottakkal alone, without counting the sales at the branches. This is the vow I am going to fulfil tonight. There is not very much more I wish for. The Arya Vaidya Sala, its branches and the establishments connected with them are now being run more or less as I had desired. All we should make certain of is not to regress from this stage.

---

[30]S.Varier: 'Addeham' (For Him, with Respect).

A number of people earn their livelihoods here in the name of drama and Kathakali. They no longer have the skills to earn their living in any other field. I must find a solution for that. I have no idea how I should do this, or what I should do. But in any case, if I have to go, I can go now with peace of mind, with satisfaction, to the other world . . .

The offering of the twelve thousand coconuts that he spoke of should have coincided with the temple festival the following year, in March 1944, the time when such offerings were usually made. But Varier insisted that it be performed in December 1943. Shinnan Menon reminded him that it was usual to have the ceremony conducted in March. 'No, let's not put it off. What if I am not alive on that day? It is a vow I made, let me honour it now, not delay it,' answered Varier.

It was a memorable night. Streamers made from palm leaves, clusters of flowers and fruit swung beneath a canopy of white and red silk in the wide space in front of the Vishvambhara temple, while the artists drew the sacred drawing of the Hunter's Son. One drew his hands, another his legs, yet another his body and a fourth his face. In the green of dried manjadi leaves, in a lime-and-turmeric mixture of red, in the yellow of turmeric alone, in the white of powdered rice, in the black of powdered charcoal, he took shape, the beautiful son of Shiva and Parvathi, born in the forest: black-bearded, armed with a bow and arrow, wearing jewels around his neck, his waist and arms, with a crown on his head and anger flashing in his reddened, protruding eyes.

Musicians played the ilathalam, chengala and nandurni and sang to their rhythms in praise of the beautiful prince: the song of his birth, his rise to fame and his superhuman feats. The chenda, the horns, the edakka and the conch joined them, while the caparisoned elephants waited, stamping their feet, the music echoing around them. Until the other self of the Hunter's

Son, the velichappadu, the possessed oracle, came out on his low wooden stool and slowly started to erase the coloured form on the ground. Suddenly, he stopped moving, began to pick up coconuts, one by one, from the huge pile of twelve thousand perfectly matured coconuts heaped up on the ground beside him and threw them, one with each hand, while the chendas thudded, their cadences mounting faster and faster while his hands swung swiftly, right, left, right, left, in perfect time . . .

When the pile of coconuts was exhausted, the velichappadu began to move again, gradually erasing the drawing on the ground until it had disappeared completely.

29 December 1943

The offering of the twelve thousand coconuts was made and everything went off very auspiciously.

What compelled Varier to fulfil that vow with such urgency? What did he think of, as the coconuts fell, one by one, and the drums throbbed faster and faster? There was a legend that Varier's ancestors had enshrined the Hunter's Son in the machu, the panelled granary, of the ancient Panniyinpally taravad house and worshipped him there. Did his family deity reach out through the colours and sounds of that night and lay a blessing on him, mutely acknowledging the magnitude of all he had achieved?

The year 1944 began well. The routine for the previous year described in the opening pages of his diary indicates that Varier's pace had slowed down, but there is no mention of any specific ailment or of a significant change in his habits. He taught the students as usual, spent time with the Kathakali artistes, went to the Vishvambhara temple every day to worship, was careful to eat food that was not highly spiced.

1 January 1944

Pulse—about 88—94—100. Respiration 7—8—9. Urine, specific gravity 1020°. Weight 126 lbs. No trouble. Blood pressure, systolic, 135. Diastolic, 85.

Yesterday the Natya Sangham was awarded a medal.

Pandit Hridayanath Kunsru, President of the Bharat Seva Sangh, came to Kottakkal on 5 January for treatment. Varier received him and supervised the arrangements for his stay.

As January progressed however, Varier began to feel unwell:

20 Januray 1944

Stopped unboiled buttermilk from this afternnon, taking it boiled instead.

Rice, little more than four ladles. Coffee, tea, just over three cups.

21 January

Slight stomach ache. Rice, 4 ladles. Coffee, tea, more than two cups. Taught Shareeram (Anatomy and Physiology). Felt tired. Drank tea at 7.15 p.m. Worshipped in the temple. Ramankutty came.

24 January 1944

Since digestion seems unsatisfactory, began to take a small amount of fried red chillies and ginger. But on the whole, eat less.

26 January 1944

Felt short of breath at night.

On 29 January, a Saturday, a cold day, full of mist, Varier felt distinctly uneasy.

29 January 1944

I have a suspicion that my pulse is stopping now and then. Ramankutty did not say anything.

I said I would not teach Shareeram today.

At noon temperature 94. Sleep not sound. Could not see Sankaran Kutty. Felt sad.

Had half a cup of coffee with glucose.

Letters 32.

At 8.45, I coughed a great deal and spat out a lot of phlegm.

Dr Ramankutty Varier, his niece's husband, who was in charge of the Charitable Hospital, used to examine P.S. Varier every day. He noted P.S. Varier's symptoms, thought he seemed slightly warm, prescribed a medicine. Although he did not teach his students that day, Varier asked them, strangely, to read the portion entitled 'The Future' in his report on the occasion of the Silver Jubilee of the Arya Vaidya Sala, a declaration that affirms his faith that the work he started would continue. He examined the patients who had come to see him and looked through his letters as usual.

That night, he ate very lightly and went to bed at 10.00, as he normally did. E. Sankunni Nair, who used to be an actor in the drama troupe, used to sleep just outside his bedroom at this period, in case he needed help. Sankunni Nair heard Varier coughing continually all night. He got up once to spit out phlegm. He seemed to have dozed a bit between 3.00 and 5.00 in the morning.

Sankunni Nair went into Varier's room as soon as he heard him stirring, about 5 a.m. on 30 January.

'I didn't sleep at all, Sankunni. Such a bad cough and I spat out a lot of phlegm too,' said Varier.

'Let me bring you some hot coffee quickly. It will make you feel better.'

'All right then. If you bring some, I'll drink it,' Varier answered with his usual light-hearted air. Sankunni Nair hurried down.

When he came back, his master was stretched out on the floor of the anteroom, wearing only a kaupeenam, his head facing southward, next to the brass oil lamp which he had evidently just lighted. His pen, his watch and his diary lay near his head. His glasses hung down from one ear. His left hand seemed to be examining the pulse of his right one. At first, Sankunni Nair did not feel alarmed. His master must have lighted the lamp, started to note his pulse and respiration to jot it down in the diary and suddenly fallen asleep because he had not slept all night. Sankunni Nair bent down and said, 'I've brought the coffee.' There was no answer. He took off Varier's glasses, his own hands trembling, and called his master again. There was still no answer. Suddenly frantic, Sankunni Nair rushed out, pushed open the window of the bedroom next door called out loudly and managed to wake up Easwara Varier, Kutty Varasyar's granddaughter's husband, who was asleep in the room just beyond. Easwara Varier hurriedly woke up Dr Ramankutty Varier.

Ramankutty Varier ran to P.S. Varier's room, bent down and examined him, then slumped to the ground, weeping. Sankunni Nair screamed and collapsed, unconscious.

In seconds, the house came alive to the news of death.

The bell over Varier's old bedroom in the Arya Vaidya Sala rang repeatedly, waking up the whole village.

Relatives tried to tell P.S. Varier's cousin, Lakshmi Varasyar, the news, but she was hard of hearing and did not understand them. However, she guessed that something terrible had taken place and turned in the direction everyone was going. When she arrived upstairs and saw her younger brother lying on the floor, she realized what had happened at once. The pitiful wail that arose from her tore through the hearts of everyone there. Lakshmi Varasyar lived another four years, but after that terrible day, no one ever saw her smile. She and Sankunni had grown up side by side. He had been with her all her life and she could not imagine that he could have gone as he did.

Thousands filed into his sitting room in Kailasamandiram that day to pay him homage. A costly red silk that the Samoothiri of Kozhikode had once bought in Kashi and gifted to Varier, covered his body, a brass oil lamp burned at his head.

But he had lighted his own oil lamp before he lay down to die, his head next to its flame. In death, as in life, he had thought ahead of everyone, and claimed the worlds that lie beyond ours as his own.

P.S. Varier's ashes rest in a niche in a little garden in the compound in front of Kailasamandiram, filled with bright flowers and dense greenery. A life-sized marble statue stands in front of the Charitable Hospital, commanding the attention of all who pass that way. But it is his indomitable spirit that permeates the very air of Kottakkal, a continuing source of inspiration to everyone who works in the establishments he founded.

So many people came to him every day of his life and each of them needed something. No one went away dissatisfied: he who was ill was treated; he who was hungry was fed; he who had no family was cared for; he who was unemployed was given gainful work; he who was illiterate was taught his letters; he who could hold a true note was taught to sing; he who could move with grace was taught to dance. Could any man have done more in the space of one short life?

22

Kottakkal Today

P.V. Rama Varier,[31] one of P.S. Varier's favourite disciples, who was manager of the Kozhikode branch of the Arya Vaidya Sala, narrates an incident from which he learnt one of the most valuable lessons in vaidyam. Once, when P.S. Varier went to Kozhikode on a weekly visit, Rama Varier had gone out to see a patient. He apologized to his teacher for having returned late, explaining that he had had to walk a few miles over fields soaked in the rain. P.S. Varier asked what he had learnt while coming back, and Rama Varier spoke at length about the symptoms of the patient he had just seen and the diagnosis he had made. His teacher listened attentively, then gently asked whether he had looked at the plants and herbs growing on either side as he walked back. Our profession is vaidyam, Varier reminded him, you must always look for medicinal plants that are useful to us, you must find out who are the vaidyans who live in the areas you pass through and

---

[31]Varier, P.V. Rama: 'My Gurunathan' in the *Souvenir of Vaidyaratnam P.S. Varier's Centenary Celebrations*.

how they find, collect and process the herbs they use in their practice. P.S. Varier's passion for vaidyam reached out to its most minute aspects and he believed that learning was a continuous process that had to be applied to every facet of life and every moment of living.

Varier carried this incessant zeal for learning and exploration into all the areas of his personal and professional life. Nothing was too difficult or too trivial for him to try out: a new way of processing a medicine, different methods of instruction for students, courses of study that sought to combine various traditions, textbooks that integrated the old and the new, variations in styles of architecture, innovative ways to stage a play, novel trends in music . . . the list was inexhaustible. He was an entrepreneur in every field of activity he was involved in and his determination to succeed was equalled only by his deep sense of commitment to whatever he did, his immense dynamism.

In his professional life, therefore, P.S. Varier was not just a vaidyan who saw his patients, diagnosed their ailments and prescribed medicines. He was anxious to ensure that they not only obtained their medicines but that the products he gave them were of the best quality. The regular system of correspondence he maintained gave patients who could not come to Kottakkal the comfort of treatment at long distance, a feature of the Arya Vaidya Sala that still operates successfully, after a hundred years.

In the social and cultural dimensions of his life, he attained a stature that not many of his contemporaries could claim. The Parama Shiva Vilasam Nataka Company and later, the P.S.V. Natya Sangham, the annual festival in the Vishvambhara temple, the reputation Kailasamandiram enjoyed of being open to vaidyans trained in any school of medicine, and to scholars and practitioners of all the performing arts: all these combined to give Kottakkal a cultural identity that added to its importance as the location of the Arya Vaidya Sala, and to Varier himself a special dignity as the person who had made this possible.

In 1944, when Varier died, it seemed difficult to imagine that Kottakkal would continue to be what it was in the absence of its dynamic founder. But the decades that followed have proved that the principles Varier had inculcated in those who worked with him were infused with a strength and power that bore the stamp of his personality and that he still remains the guiding spirit of the Arya Vaidya Sala and its offshoots.

In the years immediately following his death, it fell to P. Madhava Warrier, P.S. Varier's nephew, who was nominated the first managing trustee in his uncle's will, to carry out his uncle's wishes.

Having overcome his childhood ailments, Madhavan had qualified as an Aryavaidyan from the Patasala in Kottakkal in 1929. In 1931, he was given charge of the Vaidya Sala in Kozhikode. However, he had to go back to Kottakkal after a year and a half because of a spell of ill health. In 1932, P.S. Varier appointed him manager of the newly opened branch in Palakkad. In 1935, when Varier turned sixty-six and began to feel the need of trustworthy people around him to share his responsibilities, he summoned his nephew back to Kottakkal to assist him, and Aryavaidyan S.Varier took over in Palakkad.

Madhava Warrier had continued to fall ill during his tenure in Palakkad as well. He had an attack of smallpox soon after he joined. A few months later, the sudden death of his father shattered him emotionally. In 1933, his balance of mind was threatened and he attempted suicide many times during this distressing period. He escaped death only because he had watchful and caring people around him. Meanwhile, he was also harassed by a constant headache. P.S. Varier insisted that he go ahead with all the courses of treatment he was prescribed through this period, confident that God would not allow him to die. His unwavering faith and unremitting care saw his nephew through a succession of painful ordeals.

Once Madhavan emerged from this long period of illness, he was transformed from the slow learner he had been in childhood to an ardent and dedicated student and he engaged himself continually in courses of study throughout his short life. He had been taught Sanskrit when ill health had forced him to leave school; he later taught himself Sanskrit grammar through the well-known text, the *Laghu Panineeyam*. He then mastered English and Tamil and could write and speak both these languages with great fluency.

In 1935, Madhava Warrier married Sarojini of the Mundoor variam. This was the year his uncle called him back to Kottakkal. From this time, he was constantly with P.S. Varier, helping him with his work and gradually taking over many of his responsibilities. Varier's diaries mention him almost every day. The young man would therefore not only have observed the most minute details of the intricate network of activities that kept the vast domain of the Arya Vaidya Sala and its offshoots running smoothly, he would also have gained a deep insight into the way P.S. Varier handled each aspect of his multifaceted life.

When Varier died and Madhava Warrier took over as the first managing trustee, his aunt, Lakshmi Varasyar, pointed to P.S. Varier's sandals and asked her young nephew never to neglect to pay his respects to them. The meetings of the new trust were always held in the presence of these sandals.

From the beginning of his tenure, Madhava Warrier proved an extremely able administrator. He opened a dairy farm which produced high quality milk and ghee to be used for the processing of medicines and installed machines to extract oil. An AC generator was installed in 1949 in the factory of the Arya Vaidya Sala. Twelve grinders were installed in 1952. Pipes were laid to provide running water. He had a hostel built for the students of the Patasala. He completed the construction of the Golden Jubilee Memorial Nursing Home, which has family blocks as well as double and single rooms, all of which are equipped with modern amenities.

Apart from all the improvements he made in the establishments under his care, the income from the sale of medicines increased from Rs 1,29,424 in 1942 to Rs 10,30,670 in 1952. New branches of the Arya Vaidya Sala were opened in Tirur (1945) and Erode (1947). Toxicology was introduced as a subject of study in the Patasala. Madhava Warrier was an excellent and painstaking teacher himself and taught nervous disorders in the Patasala. By nature, he was a man who pondered deeply on things—indeed, his friends attributed his constant headaches to this inclination for excessive thinking.

Madhava Warrier decided to celebrate the Golden Jubilee of the Arya Vaida Sala on a very grand scale. A life-sized marble statue of P.S. Varier was ordered for the occasion from Nagappa and Sons, Madras. Madhava Warrier had always felt that vaidyans from all over the country needed to meet often and discuss current trends if aryavaidyam was to progress. He decided to invite the All India Ayurveda Congress to hold its thirty-ninth conference in Kottakkal to coincide with the Golden Jubilee celebrations, scheduled for 5,6 and 7 January 1954. His invitation was accepted and he went ahead with preparations for the function. In December 1953, Madhava Warrier decided to visit Bombay, to meet Pandit Shiv Sharma, the president of the congress, and finalize the details of the conference with him. Time being short, with the jubilee hardly a month away, he thought it would be wiser to fly. Strangely, almost as if she had a premonition, this decision to fly rather than travel by train made his wife uneasy and she was so insistent on going with him that he had to agree. Their return flight from Bombay was routed through Nagpur. As the aircraft took off from Nagpur at dawn on 12 December, both its engines broke down. The pilot could not make a landing and the aircraft caught fire immediately. Except for the pilot, there were no survivors. The Golden Jubilee of the Arya Vaidya Sala was postponed to 6, 7 and 8 March 1954. What would have been an occasion of great rejoicing was shadowed by the terrible grief of this tragic event. Gentle, thoughtful, considerate, Madhava Warrier had been deeply loved by all who worked with him.

Madhava Warrier's younger brother, P. Krishna Warrier (P.K. Warrier), who had been co-opted as a trustee in 1945, when Rao Bahadur P.K. Varier resigned, succeeded him and is the present managing trustee and chief physician of the Arya Vaidya Sala. During the forty-seven years he has held office, major strides have been made in the progress of every wing of the Vaidya Sala and its associate concerns. The trust board functioning now with P.K. Warrier at the helm includes P. Raghava Varier, U.E. Warrior, Dr N.S. Unnikrishnan, N.M. Vijayan, C.A. Varier and K. Balakrishna Kurup. The first five are members of the two tavazhis of the Panniyinpally family, while C.A. Varier and K. Balakrishna Kurup, I.A.S. (Retd.) have been associated with the Arya Vaidya Sala for many years.

P.K. Warrier's charismatic qualities, his dedication to research and his skill and experience as a physician have made him a figure of international repute. He has a long list of awards and honours: the Fellowship of the National Academy of Indian Medicine in 1987, a Doctorate (M.D., M.A.) from the Medicina Alternativa at Copenhagen, the title of 'Ayurved Maharshi' conferred by the All India Ayurvedic Congress, the Padma Sri awarded by the President of India in 1999, the D. Litt. of the Calicut University in 1999, the Bhoopalman Singh Special Award (SAARC level) from Kathmandu, the Millenium Gold Medal of the Academy of Ayurveda, Vijayawada, the Dr Poulose Mar Gregorios Award-2001 and the Dhanvantari Award 2001. He is a member of many important organizations: the Advanced Centre of Ayurveda in NIMHANS, Bangalore; the Scientific Advisory Committee under the Central Council for Research in Ayurveda and Siddha (CCRAS); the Ayurvedic Pharmacopoeia Committee; the Ayurveda, Siddha and Unani Drugs Technical Advisory Board; the Governing Body and Executive Committee of the Kerala Ayurvedic Studies and Research Society, Kottakkal; the Ayurveda Advisory Committee; the Committee on Drugs Control under the Government of Kerala; the Task Force on Ayurveda and Homeopathy under the State Planning Board and the Kerala Bio-Diversity Committee. He is Project Officer of the Clinical Research Unit (CCRAS) at Kottakkal. He is President of the Kerala Unit of the All India Ayurvedic Congress, Dean of the Faculty of Ayurveda and Chairman, Board of Studies in Ayurveda of the University of Calicut. He is an Expert Member of the Spices Export Council.

Under P.K. Warrier's able administration, the institution has made giant strides. The Arya Vaidya Sala in Kottakkal is now the head office and has thirteen branches. The branch in Kozhikode was opened in 1916 and the one in Palakkad in 1932, in P.S. Varier's lifetime. After his death, branches were opened in Tirur (1946), Ernakulam (1957), Thiruvananthapuram (1959), Alwaye (1962), Madras (1968), Kannur (1975), Coimbatore (1976), New Delhi (1982), Calcutta (1996), Kottayam (1998) and Secunderabad (1999). Sales depots were opened in various towns. In addition, there are more than nine hundred agencies in India which are authorized to sell the medicines processed in Kottakkal. Medicines are transported to all these agencies from Kottakkal; they are also exported abroad.

The Platinum Jubilee Ward was opened in 1979 By Morarji Desai, the then prime minister. The Adi Sankara Block, built in 1989 to accommodate the growing number of in-patients, was inaugurated by Sringeri Sankaracharya. The Centenary Block was opened by T. Sivadasa Menon in 1999. In spite of all this, there is always a long waiting list of patients seeking accommodation.

A hospital was inaugurated in New Delhi by President
K.R. Narayanan, in October 2000. It is the only unit in India
other than the one at Kottakkal which administers courses of
Ayurvedic treatment unique to Kerala. Apart from offering
advice and treatment to out-patients, it has provision for fifty
in-patients. The Delhi hospital also offers a facility that is quite
unique: out-patients are allowed to register for a course of
treatment that lasts an hour a day, go home and report the
next day for the next session of treatment.

After the formation of the Kerala state, an updated, unified
syllabus was introduced in the Ayurvedic College for a Diploma
in Ayurvedic Medicine (D.A.M.). A degree course, Bachelor of
Ayurvedic Medicine (B.A.M.) was started in 1972. A post-
graduate course in mental diseases was started in 2001.

More than 900 out-patients come every day to the Charitable
Hospital started in 1924—the queues start forming before
sunrise. About 160 in-patients a day receive free accommodation,
food, medicines and treatment. It has a Panchakarma Ward—
Panchakarma comprises five procedures of vamanam, (emesis),
virechanam (purgation), nasyam (errhines), vasti (medicated
enema) and rakthamoksham (blood-letting)—which administers
expensive courses of treatment like dhara, pizhichil and
navarakkizhi, which are unique to Kerala, free of cost to poor
patients. A maternity ward was opened in 1960. In 1966, the
hospital opened a clinical research ward with 20 beds, where
research studies are conducted in collaboration with the Central
Council for Research in Ayurveda and Siddha on in-patients
who suffer from the peptic ulcer group of diseases. The
objective is to find out methods of treatment other than
surgery that can be effective without being too expensive.
There is a poison treatment ward which specializes in the
treatment of patients who have been bitten by snakes. Studies
are being made on cancer and rheumatoid arthritis as well. A
programme on palliative care and gastroenteritis is being

conducted in collaboration with the Calicut Medical College.

There are around twelve persons now engaged in full-time and five in part-time research activity. Two joint ventures were started in 1998. The first is a collaborative research programme on bioactive molecules and allied fields conducted by the Arya Vaidya Sala and the Council for Scientific and Industrial Research (CSIR) of the Government of India. The second is a joint effort to standardize raw herbs, classical medicines and manufacturing processes undertaken by the Indian Institute of Chemical Technology of Hyderabad with the support of the Department of Science and Technology of the Government of India. Research studies are being done on medicinal herbs and a team working in collaboration with the International Development Research Centre (IDRC), Canada, studied twenty endangered species and published research papers and a book entitled *Some Important Medicinal Plants of Western Ghats, India: A Profile*. S.R. Iyer (Iyer Master) who used to be the factory manager, initiated research on medicinal plants in the late seventies. This project was developed and published in 1993 as a five-volume treatise entitled *Medicinal Plants of India—A Compendium of 500 Species* (Orient Longman, 1993).

The Arya Vaidya Samajam, under whose charge the original Patasala established by P.S. Varier functioned, was dissolved in 1976 and a new body called the Kerala Ayurvedic Studies and Research Society was formed, with representatives from the central and state governments and from the Arya Vaidya Sala. The Patasala, now known as the Vaidyaratnam P.S. Varier Ayurvedic College, functions under this body and is affiliated to Calicut University. The Ayurvedic College celebrated its Golden Jubilee in 1968 and a new building was inaugurated at the time.

In 1948, a new kitchen with thirty units was built in the Arya Vaidya Sala so that production could be increased to meet the growing demand for medicines. Grinders were installed in the fifties to grind powders and tablets. A 1.5-ton capacity steam boiler installed in 1967 replaced firewood and coconut fibre as fuel in the factory. The present installed capacity is 15 TPH.

A new factory was set up at Kanjikode in the Palakkad District in 1987. The factory at Kottakkal has about a hundred steam-jacketed steam pans and steam drug boilers; another thirty-five are in use at the Kanjikode factory. Electro-mechanical equipment is now used for almost all processing activities. Fully automated filling lines were installed in the seventies in Kottakkal and in 1987 in Kanjikode to wash, dry, fill, seal, and label bottles. The procedures for making tablets were mechanized in 1987. Kashayams (aqueous extracts) are now prepared in the form of tablets. Innovative techniques are employed to convert kashayams that taste bitter to a more palatable tablet form. Trials are now in progress for the conversion of bhasmas (powders) to capsule form. Stainless steel vessels replaced wooden vats by the late seventies for the preparation of liquid medicines like arishtams and asavams. The R&D wing of the Arya Vaidya Sala is responsible for quality control and for evolving techniques of modernization.

Medicinal plants and herbs are being scientifically cultivated in estates in Kanhirapuzha and Kottapuram in the Palakkad district. There is an eight-acre Herb Garden in Kottakkal where more than a thousand scientifically identified medicinal plant species, including some very valuable and rare ones, are cultivated for demonstration. The IDRS–AVS project on endangered medicinal plants is being conducted here.

The publication department publishes books, reference manuals and pamphlets on Ayurveda and related topics and occasionally, attakathas, the performance-texts for Kathakali. In August 1987, a bilingual quarterly called the *Arya Vaidyan*, a successor to the *Dhanvanthari* magazine, was started with Dr N.V. Krishnankutty Warrier as its chief editor.

Many of the younger members of the immediate and extended Panniyinpally family work in Kottakkal, not only as Aryavaidyans and doctors trained in western medicine but as experts in various departments—administration, finance, computers and so on.

The P.S.V. Natya Sangham now has its living quarters near the Venkitta Thevar temple and continues to stage performances and train artistes. Stipends are offered to trainees as an incentive and care is taken to adhere to the traditional Kalluvazhi style of Kathakali. New stories have been written for their repertoire. The Natya Sangham has performed all over India and in erstwhile West Germany, Denmark, Belgium, Italy, Switzerland, Indonesia, Malaysia, Singapore, China and Korea.

An annual event of great importance is held at Kottakkal on the death anniversary of P.S. Varier, Founder's Day. An Ayurveda seminar is conducted on this occasion at a national level. A thesis competition is held in which all students and professionals can participate. The thesis papers which are read on this occasion are collected and published in the seminar report. Guest speakers are invited to give two speeches: the P.S. Varier Commemorative Speech on a general topic and the P.S. Varier Memorial Speech with relevance to the founder and his achievements. The Arya Vaidya Sala also participates in many seminars and conferences at the national and international levels.

At eighty, P.K. Warrier continues to devote his time and energy tirelessly to discussing and carrying out further improvements and innovations and planning new schemes. With the support and help of the dedicated trust board, the Arya Vaidya Sala not only prospers as an institution in itself, but has proved that Ayurveda can adapt itself to a changing society and provide comfort to everyone. Ayurveda is not only very highly thought of now, it is greatly sought after by all sections of Indian society and the world as a dependable and benign system of health care.

Progress can be charted in so many ways: by facts and figures, awards and trophies, the evolution of modern techniques. In Kottakkal it is measured even today in terms of one man's dream and the single-mindedness with which he gave that dream shape and substance.

Index